HYDROGEN IMMUNOTHERAPY MAKES CANCER

DISAPPEAR

Advice from a Japanese Authority on Immuno-Oncology about how to Enhance Your Immunity Swiftly and Build a Robust Body

Junji Akagi

Can Hydrogen Be Used to Eliminate Cancer and Extend the Remaining Lifespan?

Astonishing Clinical Cases

K·H (33 years old) ♀ (P.134)

- ### Ovarian Cancer (Stage 4)
  Hyperthermia Therapy + Low-Dose Antineoplastic Drugs + Hydrogen + Opdivo®

CT (Computed Tomography) Images

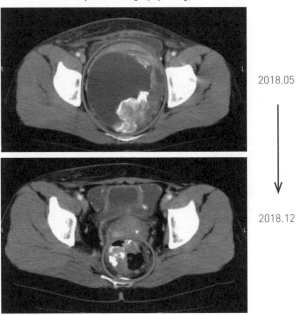

2018.05

2018.12

Tumor Size (see red circle)

112.93X107.07mm → 39.27X37.63mm

RECIST* 65.2% Reduction

*RECIST is the acronym of Response Evaluation Criteria in Solid Tumors.

H·S (62 years old) ♀ (P.135)

- ## Lung Cancer (Stage 4)
  Hyperthermia Therapy + Low-Dose Antineoplastic
  Drugs + Hydrogen + Opdivo®

PET (Positron Emission Tomography)-CT Images

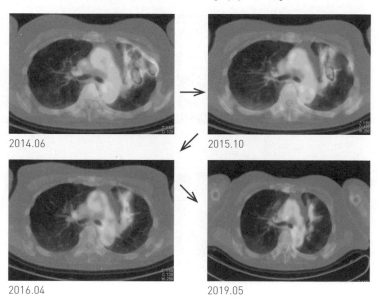

2014.06

2015.10

2016.04

2019.05

Tumor Size (shown in red)

The tumors found in mediastinal lymph nodes and the pelvis are
almost cured.

K·M (46 years old) ♀ (P.137)

● Breast Cancer (Stage 4)

Hyperthermia Therapy + Low-Dose Antineoplastic Drugs
+ Hydrogen + Opdivo®

PET-CT Images

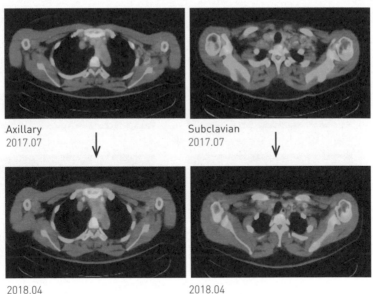

Axillary
2017.07

Subclavian
2017.07

2018.04

2018.04

Tumor Size (shown in red)

The images show that the axillary tumors are almost gone.

T·K (77 years old) ♀ (P.139)

- ● Colon Cancer (Recurrence)
  Hyperthermia Therapy + Low-Dose Antineoplastic
  Drugs + Hydrogen + Opdivo®

PET-CT Images

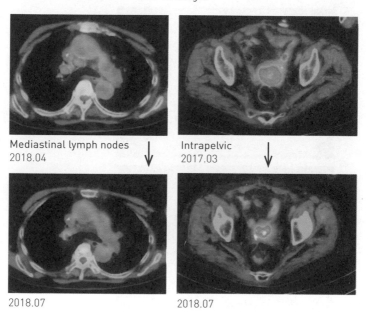

Mediastinal lymph nodes
2018.04

Intrapelvic
2017.03

2018.07

2018.07

Tumor Size (shown in red)

The tumors found in mediastinal lymph nodes and the pelvis are
significantly decreased in size.

K·K (69 years old) ♂ (P.141)

- ## Ureteral Cancer (Stage 4)
  Hyperthermia Therapy + Low-Dose Antineoplastic Drugs
  + Hydrogen + Opdivo®

CT Images

2016.10

2017.11

Tumor Size (indicated with "+")

81.94X50.18mm → 53.76 X 41.90mm
RECIST 34.4% Reduction.

T·M (53 years old) ♀ [P.142]

- ## Breast Cancer (Recurrence)
  Hyperthermia Therapy + Low-Dose Antineoplastic
  Drugs + Hydrogen

CT Images

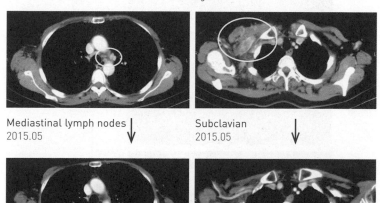

Mediastinal lymph nodes ↓
2015.05

Subclavian ↓
2015.05

2017.11

2017.11

Tumor Size (see yellow circle)

The images show that the circled tumors found in mediastinal
lymph nodes and the subclavian region have disappeared.

M·M (81 years old) ♀ [P.146]

- ## Pancreatic Cancer (Stage 4)
  Hyperthermia Therapy + Low-Dose Antineoplastic Drugs
  + Hydrogen + Opdivo®

PET-CT Images

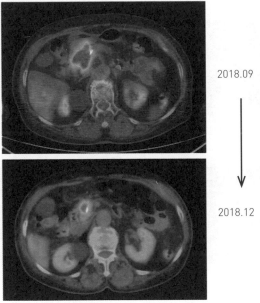

2018.09

2018.12

Tumor Size (indicated with "+")

RECIST 52.4% Reduction.

Hydrogen Immunotherapy Makes Cancer Disappear

By Junji Akagi

Hydrogen Immunotherapy Makes Cancer Disappear
By Junji Akagi

SUISO GAS DE GAN WA KIERU!?
Copyright © TATSUMI PUBLISHING CO., LTD. 2019
© JUNJI AKAGI
English translation rights arranged with TATSUMI PUBLISHING CO., LTD.
through Japan UNI Agency, Inc., Tokyo

Published in Taiwan in 2021 by China Times Publishing Company,
7F, 240, Hoping West Road, Section 3, Taipei 108019, Taiwan
www.readingtimes.com.tw

ISBN 978-957-13-9719-1
Printed in Taiwan

Can Oxy-hydrogen Be Used to Treat COVID-19?

By Dr. He-Chang Kuo, M.D.,
Professor of the School of Medicine of
Chang Gung University

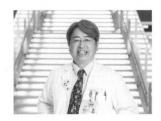

As COVID-19 continues its reign over the world and spreads rapidly across 100+ countries, the number of confirmed cases and death toll has been rising steadily, especially in the western world. The development of specific medicines and vaccines has been actively pursued in every country, but concrete treatment measures still remain unclear. At the time of publishing, experts in China have put oxy-hydrogen equipment to use as a first-line adjuvant therapy for COVID-19 and received excellent responses. It just so happened that the new book of Dr. Junji Akagi, who has gained extensive clinical experience and released myriads of research articles in Japan, was planned to be translated and published in Taiwan. It is my pleasure and honor to write this recommendation and to act as a reviewer together with Dr. Ming-Hsien

Huang, Vice Superintendent of E-Da Cancer Hospital. I believe the launch of this book will be a great drive to the establishment of the "Taiwan Association for the Promotion of Molecular Hydrogen."

From my professional point of view as an international immunologist, the application of oxy-hydrogen in the treatment of COVID-19 may not only reduce symptoms associated with difficulty breathing, but also exhibit critical anti-inflammatory effect. Taiwan has mastered the international key technology of oxy-hydrogen equipment and helped in the fight against the global pandemic by providing such equipment free of charge for frontline healthcare. I myself have been ranked as the No. 1 Asian expert on Kawasaki Disease. Since our domestic Kawasaki Disease research team reported the influence of free radicals on cardiovascular condition in patients with Kawasaki Disease in 2002 (J. Pediatr. 2002 Oct ; 141(4): 560-5.), it has been suggested that the elimination or neutralization of free radicals is highly beneficial to the treatment of Kawasaki Disease. From then on, we have been working hard to investigate the effective free radical scavenger.

In Japan, the use of hydrogen in healthcare and treatment has been ongoing for more than a decade. I have been following this area since I read a paper written by Japanese authors as early as 2007, illustrating the suitability of applying hydrogen in health maintenance and as a complementary role in disease treatment in *Nature Medicine* (Nature Medicine. 2007 Jun; 13(6): 688-94.). In addition, the recent article presented by Dr. Akagi in *Oncology Reports* (Oncol Rep. 2019 Jan; 41(1):301-311. SCI IF:3.041), demonstrating the improvement of rectal cancer prognosis with the use of hydrogen, has even strengthened our confidence in bringing hydrogen into clinical use.

At exhibitions of medicine and biotechnology held in the last two years, I came to know about oxy-hydrogen generators. I was surprised that nearly all of the relevant technology adopted overseas has originally derived from Taiwan. For so many years, I have always wanted to perform large-scale clinical studies on allergic diseases and Kawasaki Disease with the goal of using hydrogen-neutralized free radicals in adjuvant therapy for pediatric patients. It is my sincere wish that increased support may be given by the associated authorities to create a local research database in Taiwan and to keep up with the study progress of Japan and the others.

I would like to thank Dr. Akagi for compiling and

sharing these clinical cases. We intend to translate this compilation to expand public benefits. Certainly, research is the foundation of medical advancement. Dr. Akagi has been contributing to the progression of hydrogen medicine through clinical trials and publications in international journals. Now, he has even written a popular science book to share his clinical data and analyses, a demonstration of a true spirit of generous giving. Under the challenges brought on by the COVID-19 pandemic, it is exciting to see the release of a book describing hydrogen therapy in English version. I am looking forward to the publication of this new book and the succeeding establishment of the related societies, as well as the promotion of molecular hydrogen medicine and future healthcare.

Prof. & Dr. He-Chang Kuo

· Professor at the School of Medicine of Chang Gung University
· Director of Kawasaki Disease Center of Kaohsiung Chang Gung Memorial Hospital
· No. 1 Asian expert on Kawasaki Disease ranked by Expertscape
· Director general of Taiwan Association for the Promotion of Molecular Hydrogen
· Professor of the Dept. of Pediatric Internal Medicine, Kaohsiung Chang Gung Memorial Hospital
· Fellow of the American Academy of Allergy Asthma and Immunology (FAAAAI)
· Director general of Kawasaki Disease Taiwan

Does Hydrogen Make Cancer Disappear? —— My Opinion about Oxy-hydrogen Therapy

By Dr. Ming-Hsien Huang,
Vice Superintendent of E-Da Cancer Hospital

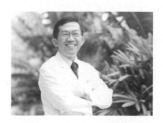

The author, Dr. Junji Akagi, is Superintendent of Tamana Regional Health Medical Center in Japan. After discovering the phenomenon of immune cell activation induced by hydrogen, Dr. Akagi has combined Opdivo® with a medical hydrogen generator made in Japan to conduct clinical trials on terminal cancer patients. More than 400 patients have received the treatment since 2016. It has been shown by the study data that oxy-hydrogen inhalation helps to increase Opdivo® response rate and triggers immune cell activation in cancer patients. The study outcome has been published by Dr. Akagi in oncology journals in the US, UK, and Japan. Moreover, Dr. Akagi has participated in several medical seminars in Japan, China, and Taiwan, and presented the topic of "Cancer Immunotherapy—the Effect of Combined

Treatment of Opdivo® and Hydrogen," which has gathered the attention of physicians and scholars from many countries, as well as my research interest. The topic has gathered the attention of physicians and scholars from many countries, as well as my research interest. Therefore, I have begun performing a clinical study investigating the influence of hydrogen inhalation on the side effects of targeted therapy for lung cancer at E-Da Cancer Hospital in Taiwan since the autumn of 2019.

There is an increasing number of literature demonstrating the diverse bioactivities inducible by oxy-hydrogen inhalation, which include primarily anti-inflammatory and anti-reactive oxygen species effects. Evidence has also suggested that hydrogen seems capable of mitigating the side effects of traditional chemotherapy, or inhibiting the growth of tumor cells and xenotransplanted tumors in in vitro and in vivo animal studies, indicating promising and extensive applications of hydrogen in clinical adjuvant therapy. Our study has included 20 patients with lung adenocarcinoma who have received EGFR-TKI treatment and have grade 2 to 4 dermal toxicity. Topical steroids, topical antibiotics, and oral antibiotics have been prescribed to control the side effects of dermal toxicity. The participants have been required to inhale oxy-hydrogen for at least 3 hours daily.

According to the study result, no adverse effect has been observed in any patient after 4 to 12 weeks of inhalation therapy. In addition, the papular rash arising from EGFR-TKI treatment has been dramatically reduced after oxy-hydrogen inhalation. In order to confirm whether hydrogen inhalation lowers the dermal toxicity associated with EGFR-TKI, it is necessary to expand the study scale in the future.

The probability of developing cancer has increased significantly with the extension of the average life expectancy. This book is the first collection of the comments made by a Japanese immuno-oncologist on "hydrogen immunotherapy." During the release of its Chinese version in Taiwan, Dr. Akagi has established an immunotherapy center in Kumamoto, Japan, featuring the service of combination therapy of Opdivo® and hydrogen. From the perspective of cancer treatment, Dr. Akagi has presented an abundance of empirical data associated with oxy-hydrogen therapy to offer a new treatment position to the world.

Prof. & Dr. Ming-Hsien Huang

Specialty: Diagnosis and treatment of lung cancer, asthma, chronic obstructive pulmonary disease, geriatric medicine, and clinical cytology

Certification: Internal medicine specialist, chest medicine specialist

Education: M.D. from the School of Medicine, Kaohsiung Medical University, M.D./Ph.D from Tokyo Medical University

Experience:

· Vice Superintendent of the Dept. of Internal Medicine at E-Da Cancer Hospital (incumbent)
· Research fellow at Mayo Clinic
· Professor of Internal Medicine of Kaohsiung Medical University
· Director of the Dept. of Internal Medicine, Vice Superintendent, and Acting Superintendent at Kaohsiung Medical University Hospital
· Director general of Taiwan Elderly Care and Health Promotion Association (incumbent)
· Attending physician of Dept. of Chest Medicine at E-Da Cancer Hospital (incumbent)
· Research fellow at University of Arkansas
· Director of the Dept. of Medical Sociology and Social Work and Dept. of Respiratory Therapy at Kaohsiung Medical University
· Director of the Division of Geriatrics at Kaohsiung Medical University Hospital

Persistence Turns what Seemed Unbelievable Yesterday into the Convention of Tomorrow

By Dr. Wen-Chang Lin, Ph.D.,
Chairman of Epoch Energy Technology Co.,
and Ota Hydrogen Biotech

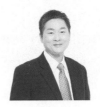

I have studied oxy-hydrogen equipment for more than 30 years, and the one thing I care about most in the usage of hydrogen is safety. Over the past twenty years, hydrogen has been applied to different types of technology industries. Starting from 2010, I spent 4 years working as a visiting professor at Kanazawa University in Japan, and began to study hydrogen applications in the human body with local scholars. Afterwards, Epoch Energy Technology Co., a long-standing oxy-hydrogen equipment manufacturer, decided to invest in this field. Its business focus was directed towards healthcare and medicine markets subsequent to the patent licensing of our *hydrogen generator* in Taiwan in 2012. Since there has been no relevant medical equipment in the past, *our hydrogen generator* has been promoted as a healthcare product featured to offer anti-oxidation and anti-aging effects through the eradication of free radicals. In addition to patents acquired in Taiwan, Japan, China, and many other countries, *our hydrogen generator* has been awarded the Symbol of National Quality among other products designed for long-term care.

Mr. Takaaki Arisawa, Chairman of Helix Japan Inc., is my business partner in Japan. After using *our hydrogen*

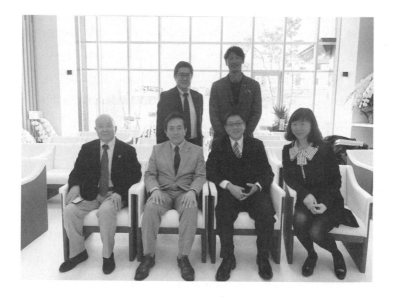

On the front from left to right: Mr. Takaaki Arisawa, Dr. Junji Akagi, Dr. Wen-Chang Lin, and Ms. Ssu-Hung Cheng from Helix Japan.
On the back from left to right: Mr. Yukio Tsuyama from Helix Japan, and Mr. Seiichiro Maki, former Japanese football player.

generator, Mr. Arisawa, who had experienced great improvement in his general health, had the intuition that "oxy-hydrogen healthcare" would become a high potential candidate in the health market. Thus, he determined to pass down the construction company he founded sixty years earlier to his offspring, and created Helix Japan Inc. at the age of 80 to fully engage in the popularization of the *hydrogen generator*. Moreover, Mr. Arisawa, a beneficiary of oxy-hydrogen healthcare, was willing to obtain the Japanese dealership for local manufacturing at a cost of several hundred millions of yen. Nowadays, oxy-hydrogen healthcare is provided in many hospitals, clinics, and massage centers in Japan, and oxy-hydrogen is mostly used as adjuvant cancer treatment in clinical medicine. Recently, I have been collaborating with the University of Tokyo in further exploring the advantages of oxy-hydrogen healthcare in human health. Apart from cancer, for example, clinical research on dementia is planned. A previous study conducted by the University of Yamanashi to examine the effect of fatigue reduction resulted from oxy-hydrogen healthcare after high-intensity exercise has also shown positive outcomes.

In 2016, I was honored to provide professional introduction of hydrogen and the quantification of different gases to Mr. Arisawa and Dr. Junji Akagi. After assessing practical requirements, Dr. Akagi decided to set up the starting point for an innovative treatment by combining the ET-100 oxy-hydrogen equipment with immunotherapy. On February 1, 2020, as the inventor of the *hydrogen generator*, I was invited to attend the opening ceremony of the immunotherapy center led by Dr. Akagi in Japan. During the visit, it was incredibly thrilling and touching to see ET-100 deployed in every room of the facility. The scene reminded me of what Dr. Chao-long Chen, also known as "the father of liver transplant in Asia," once wrote in a book he gave me more than a decade ago, "persistence turns what seemed unbelievable yesterday into the convention of tomorrow."

Hydrogen Immunotherapy makes cancer disappear is a bestseller in Japan. The complete case data and treatment schemes studied and recorded by Dr. Akagi are surely great contribution to oxy-hydrogen applications in the future of medicine. This is a book definitely worth recommending.

Dr. Wen-Chang Lin, Ph.D

Experience:
- Chairman of Epoch Energy Technology Co.
- Chairman of Ota Hydrogen Biotech
- Ph.D. from the Postgraduate Institute of Mechanics and Precision Engineering, National Kaohsiung University of Science and Technology
- M.M from the Postgraduate Institute of Hi-Tech Management, University of South Australia

Declaration: This book is simply the translated version of its Japanese original. The intention is to present the clinical cases shared by the author. The before-and-after comparison is merely part of the presentation of individual cases, which should not be deemed as the indication of clinical effectiveness or treatment advice, or the representation of the stance of the publisher or any professionals recommending this book.

Foreword

"Goodness! The tumor in the lymph nodes was gone! We actually have just started the treatment two weeks ago..." As a specialist in immuno-oncology, I have been treating cancer for over three decades. During these thirty years, various cancer therapies have been developed with the advances in the field of medicine. Although they may be helpful to some patient groups, we are still lacking a single treatment that has been recognized to be effective to most people.

I have been attempting day after day, as a doctor, to mitigate the suffering and to prolong the lives of my patients by all means. In my career, I have never seen any patient experiencing such a speedy recovery in just two weeks. Frankly speaking, when Ms. K·H, 68 years old, came in to our hospital two weeks ago, I even thought to myself, "this poor lady may not be able to leave this place alive." That's exactly how serious her condition was.

The recurrence of her breast cancer had metastasized to her bones, liver, and cervical lymph nodes, generating a substantial mass on the right side of her jaw. I knew

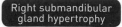

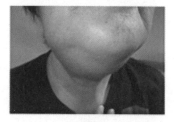

CT shows lymph node metastases

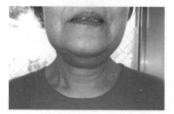

Two weeks later

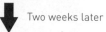

The swelling of the lymph nodes was gone after the application of hydrogen for two weeks.

Ms. K·H had experienced a breast cancer recurrence and metastases to cervical lymph nodes, resulting in her swollen jaw. After adding hydrogen to her treatment, the swelling disappeared rapidly within two weeks.

from my previous experience that she was in a critical condition, but I wanted to save her still. This desire prompted me to try on something that was introduced to me not long ago—hydrogen, something that is ubiquitous in nature and present in us all.

In my usual practice, I use immunotherapy to treat cancer, and my treatment protocol basically consists of hyperthermia therapy, low-dose antineoplastic drugs, and Opdivo® (the medicine used in cancer immunotherapy). In Ms. K·H's case, by the addition of hydrogen, I was deeply surprised to see the remission of her hypertrophic right submandibular gland in just a short period of two weeks.

Since January 2015, Ms. K·H had continued to take antineoplastic drugs, such as Avastin® + paclitaxel, Avastin® + Abraxane®, and Halaven® for treatment of her recurrent breast cancer, but the value of the tumor marker CA 15-3 had been increasing steadily. Until July 6, 2016, the value rose up to 1630 accompanying her lymph node swelling. This soaring trend is specific to patients with breast cancer. Normally, the value of the tumor marker CA 15-3 should be lower than 31.3. An abnormal level this high may be reflective of the potential presence of multiple metastases to bones and liver. Nevertheless, in two weeks after receiving the combined treatment of immunotherapy and hydrogen, the right submandibular gland hypertrophy had disappeared, and Ms. K·H was discharged in good health. On August 3, approximately one month later, the CA 15-3 value had decreased to 1132.

Before I started treating Ms. K·H, I was introduced by one of my friends to a hydrogen generator, and it was suggested that "hydrogen is useful in cancer treatment." I was not persuaded initially, but after I realized that hydrogen does not result in potential explosion hazard and is beneficial to the human body in many ways, I couldn't help thinking, "perhaps this is something worth trying." Afterwards I witnessed Ms. K·H's case, which brought me to an idea that "hydrogen may become one of the great promises for cancer treatment in the future."

Consequently, I have begun to perform ongoing research and established *hydrogen immunotherapy* at last. **This is the first attempt in the world to treat cancer with hydrogen**, and we have successfully cured more than 400 patients to significantly prolong the remaining lifespan of many end-stage or recurrent cancer patients. In addition, I published my article in the British academic journal, *Oncology Reports*, and received considerable attention globally. In December 2018, I gave a speech about "the advent of the application of immunotherapy for advanced cancer—combined immunotherapy" at the 6th World Integrative Medicine Congress held in Shanghai, China (where 2,500 doctors participated). In May 2019, a group of 40 doctors from China attended the event hosted by the Society for Integrative Medicine Japan at Aichi Medical University. Also, in mid-June of the same year, I departed for Guangzhou, China to attend a relevant event.

Written in the above-mentioned background, this book documents the details of the unprecedented *hydrogen*

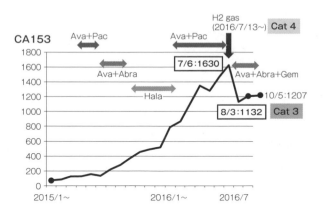

The steadily rising value of the tumor marker showed a dramatic drop.
The value of the tumor marker CA 15-3 had increased abnormally because of breast cancer recurrence. Typically, the normal value should be lower than 31.3, whereas it reached to 1630 when Ms. K·H was presented with the swollen lymph node and then decreased to 1132 within a month of the application of hydrogen therapy.

immunotherapy in the world. While the standard of care, including antineoplastic drugs and radiotherapy, has failed to cure cancer and become a hopeless option by physicians, I wish to inform the distressed or exhausted patients and families of a potentially promising treatment approach, the mechanism and case reports of which are covered in this book. I think, even if you have been told, "there is nothing we can do for you now," or asked, "are you willing to consider palliative care?" it would be truly a blessing to learn that there is still hope of survival.

† Reviewers' comment:The Hydrogen mentioned in this book is referred to as the mixture of hydrogen and oxygen, rather than pure hydrogen gas.

Table of Contents

Chapter 2

Patients Have No Choice

Chapter 3

Immune Deficiency Is an Obstacle to the Success of Antineoplastic drugs and Radiotherapy

Chapter 4

Curing End-Stage Cancer Patients With Hydrogen

Chapter 7 ————————————————————————

Hydrogen Prolongs Healthy Lifespan by 10 Years

Chapter 8 ———————————————————————

The Era of Customized Treatment Approaches

Chapter 1

Some Cancer May Disappear, while Some May Not

Rapid-and Slow-Growing Cancers

Did you know that the growth rate of various carcinomas, albeit all being called by the same name as cancer, may vary based on their primary origins? Certain types of cancer, such as pancreatic cancer and cholangiocarcinoma, are difficult to detect at their early stage and fast-growing compared with other cancers. In these cases, remission is rarely seen, and significantly increased recurrence risks are observed even when the tumor is surgically removed. Poor prognosis has made close post-operative monitoring a necessity for these patients. On the other hand, thyroid cancer is a good example of slow-growing cancers. With its generally good prognosis, it has been reported that many patients have survived up to ten years in peaceful coexistence with thyroid cancer.

In 2017, cancer types shown with a higher mortality rate were inclusive of lung, colorectal, stomach, pancreatic, liver and breast cancers. Among them, colorectal cancer and breast cancer are associated with better prognosis, followed by stomach cancer and lung cancer. In contrast, pancreatic cancer is linked to substantially poorer prognosis, while liver cancer shows

a slightly less poor scenario. Prognosis is highly related to the probability of metastasis. In other words, cancers associated with good prognosis are basically non-metastatic.

Cancer Types with High Mortality in Japan

	Top 1	Top 2	Top 3	Top 4	Top 5
Male	Lung Cancer	Stomach Cancer	Colorectal Cancer	Liver Cancer	Pancreatic Cancer
Female	Colorectal Cancer	Lung Cancer	Pancreatic Cancer	Stomach Cancer	Breast Cancer
Total	Lung Cancer	Colorectal Cancer	Stomach Cancer	Pancreatic Cancer	Liver Cancer

Colorectal, stomach, and lung cancers are associated with better prognosis. Colorectal cancer, stomach cancer, and lung cancer demonstrated a better prognosis compared to the other cancer types with high mortality in 2017. (Source: Center for Cancer Control and Information Services, National Cancer Center Japan)

Moreover, the growth rate of various carcinomas may differ depending on *cancer grading* and *immunogenicity*. **The concept of cancer grading is referred to as the fact that different organs may give rise to different types of cancer cells, and the growth rate of cancer cells is primarily determined by its grading.** That is to say, a single type of cancer cells does not spread across the whole body to cause multiple diseases. Instead, cancer cells may be generated differently by the individually cancerized organs. For example, pancreatic cancer developed from cancer cells originating and proliferating in the pancreas is considered of high grading, which can be aggressive and rapidly progressing. On the contrary, thyroid cancer formed by cancer cells generating in the thyroid gland is considered of low grading, and may be equally implied as slowly progressing.

Another decisive factor is *immunogenicity*, which is correlated with the amount of antigens (cancer markers) expressed on a specific type of cancer cells and identifiable by immune cells. If the expressed antigens are easily recognized, it is highly likely that cancer cells, prior to proliferation, may be destroyed by the immune system to prevent metastasis and result in better prognosis. By contrast, in the event that early recognition of antigens is unachievable, which means that immune cells are easily evaded by cancer cells, the probability of metastasis may rise and lead to poorer prognosis.

Consequently, **cancer grading is also decided on whether malignant cells are easily identified by the immune system or not.** To put it another way, cancer cells arising from the pancreas is considered of high grading because they are hardly identified by immune cells, whereas cancer cells generating in the thyroid gland is considered of low grading because they are easily spotted by the immune system.

Cancer Development Is Contributed by Your Lifestyle

Cancer is easily formed when our immune system becomes weakened. The primary causes of low immunity are stress and lifestyle, which means one of the keys to cancer prevention lies in immune enhancement achieved by stress reduction and lifestyle correction. According to some theory, **there are 5 thousand cancer cells generated in the human body each day.** People without cancer do not exhibit any signs of illness because their immunity is strong enough to suppress cancer cell proliferation. Yet, people affected by immunodeficiency may develop cancer since their natural defense mechanisms fail to stop the reproduction of cancer cells.

Allegedly, **one in every two Japanese may suffer from cancer.** This description may be translated into a 50% of abnormal immune responses in Japanese

One in every two Japanese may suffer from cancer

The chance of having cancer in one's life

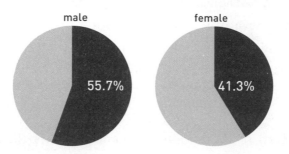

male   female

55.7%   41.3%

Living in the era in which a party of married couples may suffer from cancer
For Japanese, the current probability of cancer development is estimated to be 50%. Cancer has become one of the common illnesses in our lives, and the main cause of this is the ever changing lifestyles which have brought about the disorderly dietary style and excessive stress.

population. Starting from the 1970s, supermarkets and fast foods have begun to flourish in Japan. In the meantime, patients suffering from hay fever, ulcerative colitis, and Crohn's disease have started to increase in proportion. While these disorders are caused by an overreaction of the immune system, cancer is resulted from immune deficiency, which is at the complete opposite end of the spectrum of immune abnormality.

It has been suggested that such diseases are arisen from modern lifestyles. But in any case, dietary styles surely make the most impact on the status quo. Food products that are readily served by supermarkets and fast food restaurants contain a large amount of additives and preservatives, overconsumption of which should be avoided. Nonetheless, it is almost impossible to completely wipe them out of our lives. So what do we have to do with this?

First of all, immune enhancement is the most important thing for everyone. It is said that our body produces five thousand cancer cells per day. The maintenance of high levels of immunity may protect us against cancer development by suppressing cancer cell proliferation. In the case of patients with stage 4 cancer, immunotherapy may be helpful to strengthen the self-healing ability and to win a chance of extending survival for another 1, 3, or 5 years. We have been taking care of many stage 4 patients in our hospital, who have proven to us the utmost importance of immune enhancement during cancer treatment.

95% Cure Rate of Early Cancer

The cure rate of early cancer may vary by its

primary origin. For example, a cure rate up to 95% has been reported for stomach, colorectal, ovarian, breast, thyroid, and prostate cancers. But then, many patients have died from the early stage of pancreatic cancer and cholangiocarcinoma, with only a survival rate of 40%. These types of cancer are difficult to discover at their early stage, hence the optimal treatment window is often missed, leading to certain progression in most patients when the diagnosis is finally confirmed.

Furthermore, normally after surgery, a small amount of residual cancer cells may be detected and eliminated by immune cells. But pancreatic cancer cells may morph into patterns unrecognizable by immune cells to escape immune surveillance, resulting in instant cancer cell reproduction in most patients. Thus, it is necessary to pay close attention to the prognosis of such cases.

Advanced and Recurrent Cancer Create a Refractory Condition Within Our Bodies

Cancer treatment is strongly associated with the immune system. The leading role in immunity is played by *CD8 killer T cells* that are responsible for the detection and destruction of cancer cells. For the induction of CD8 killer T cells, it is important to apply the newly advocated concept of *cancer-immunity cycle (CIC)* described below.

Firstly, cancer cells are impaired by antineoplastic drugs or radiotherapy (Step 1 Cancer Cell Impairment) and engulfed by dendritic cells, i.e. antigen-presenting cells, (Step 2 Cancer Antigen/Tumor Marker Expression by Dendritic Cells). Lymphocytes, upon recognizing the tumor marker, produce CD8 killer T cells for cancer cell identification (Step 3 T cell Education by Dendritic Cells). T cells then move around in the bloodstream (Step 4 T cell Trafficking), reaching the tumor site (Step 5 Infiltration into the Tumor Site) to detect (Step 6 Recognition of Cancer Cells) and destroy cancer cells (Step 7 Killing of Cancer Cells). So long as every step of the CIC operates as expected, the key player—CD8 killer T cells—can be generated to eliminate cancer cells.

Nevertheless, advanced and recurrent cancer may undermine the CIC and specifically affect *PD-1* involved in Step 7. In 2018, Dr. Tasuku Honjo, Distinguished Professor of Kyoto University, was awarded the Nobel Prize for his discovery of PD-1, This news might have made the public familiar with the substance called PD-1. Usually, PD-1 is presented on the surface of CD8 killer T cells in cancer patients. The combination of PD-1 and *PD-L1* expressed on cancer cells may initiate the *immunosuppression*, preventing CD8 killer T cells from destroying cancer cells. Opdivo® is mainly used to aid in PD-L1/PD-1 blockade to relieve the immunosuppression and resume the attack launched by CD8 killer T cells against cancer cells. However, cancer cells may still secret *cytokines* to create an unsupportive environment to the CIC. Hindrance immune function and suitability for cancer proliferation are the common feature of advanced and recurrent cancer as well as the main reason why they remain refractory.

It is often said among doctors that, "cancer cells are good at disguising themselves." In stage 1 cancer, malignant cells may be removed instantly by immune cells upon exposure. In advanced or recurrent cancer, however, **cancer cells may impede the CIC while concealing the tumor marker to evade immune detection.** That is, cancer cells may bypass immune surveillance by disguising themselves as normal cells. In a sense, cancer cells are very smart. They make swift changes in order to survive. In addition, cancer cells evolve actively to produce resistance to antineoplastic drugs, waning the drug efficacy gradually. That is why cancer patients are always reminded by their doctors to "be careful of the relapse." A relapse does not occur when the immune system maintains its normal function, and a recurrence is an unfortunate but obvious indication of a weakened immune system. As a result, it is very critical to boost the immunity in advance.

Diet Therapies Are Helpful but Not Enough

There are many diet therapies, food products, and dietary supplements claiming to be effective for cancer patients, such as the Gerson therapy—emphasizing a considerable intake of vegetables—and supplements containing food extracts. However, we must admit it is extremely difficult to overcome cancer simply by means of adopting diet therapies and consuming dietary supplements. From an immunological perspective, should we assume the effectiveness of immunotherapy to be 100%, the efficacy induced by diet therapies or dietary supplements is equal to an expectation of 1% only. These methods are not baneful, of course, **but we must realize the fact that they are not powerful enough to eradicate cancer.** In fact, they are not even sufficient to stop cancer progression.

Even though some people may experience dramatic effects from diet therapies every now and then, we cannot assume they are equally effective to a number of ten thousand people. It is a very dangerous idea to conquer cancer simply through diet, and only a handful of success; have been documented in the literature so far. Anything claiming *effective for immune enhancement* should not be taken in blindly. Please bear in mind that when considering a practical treatment, it is essential to know for sure how effective it is exactly. Despite saying that, I am delighted to see the application of diet therapies or dietary supplements as adjuvant cancer treatment. Just like the association between a *treatment* and an *adjuvant*, we are supposed to figure out their respective capabilities in order to employ them accordingly.

Chapter 2

Patients Have No Choice

What Are the Three Major Types of Cancer Treatment?

Operative procedure (surgery), medication (antineoplastic drugs), and radiation therapy are commonly known as the three major types of cancer treatment. These treatment methods are described as the *standard of care* and are applicable to Japanese National Health Insurance (NHI). Normally, for stage 1 to stage 3 cancer, the basic standard of care starts from removing the cancerized organ via surgery. Successful resection is defined by the complete removal of cancer cells, whereas unsuccessful resection leave traces of cancer cells and may result in treatment failure in many cases.

Following surgery, the patient may have to receive antineoplastic drugs or radiotherapy. But these measures are not useful for clearing advanced cancer surviving after unsuccessful resection or relapsing postoperatively. To wipe out cancer cells thoroughly, it is necessary to conduct treatment from a fundamental level, which means to spy on cancer cells with the immune system in order to prevent any possible reproduction of the invisibly malignant remnants.

However, antineoplastic drugs and radiotherapy may undermine the fundamental treatment by damaging the immune system altogether with cancer cells. In particular, the standard dose of antineoplastic drugs which is calculated by the patient's body weight and body surface area, is intended to kill the maximum amount of cancer cells. It simply destroys cancer cells along with immune cells without giving any thought to the impact on the immune system. The truth is, **we could have used our own immunity to achieve self-healing in the first place, but the state of immunodeficiency inflicted by our choice of cancer treatment has made the battle more difficult.**

During the course of radiotherapy, the lesion is exposed to radiation from different angles. The advancement of recent techniques allows the radiation beam to be focused on the tumor site, but the skin surface of the exposed area may still be burned. Undoubtedly, a treatment as destructive as such cripples the immune function of the human body.

A well-functioning cancer-immunity cycle (CIC) is essential to cancer treatment. Thus, antineoplastic drugs must be firstly administered to damage cancer cells and to initiate the CIC. Although the destruction of cancer cells by antineoplastic drugs or radiotherapy is required at the beginning, a catastrophic level of impairment should be avoided to keep the immune system integrated. A recent saying goes, "immunogenic cell death is the prerequisite for immune induction." In other words, **to activate the immune system, it is important to kill a sufficient but not necessarily massive amount of cancer cells.**

Meanwhile, please note that treatments designed for immune enhancement are indispensable. As a specialist working in immuno-oncology for more than 30 years, I am confident to assert the essentiality of the immunity in cancer treatment. Furthermore, the fact that Professor Tasuku Honjo won the 2018 Nobel Prize in Physiology or Medicine for his research on Opdivo®—an anticancer immunotherapy agent—has seemed to be a declaration to the world that **the immunity is the key to cancer eradication.** To my delight, the importance of the immune system in cancer treatment has gradually gained extensive attention through Professor Tasuku Honjo's remarkable accomplishment.

What Is the "Standard" for the "Standard of Care"?

The so-called standard of care is referred to as treatment methods applicable to Japanese NHI, which are inclusive of surgery, antineoplastic drugs, and radiotherapy. The criterion for the standard of care is based solely on the standard of *killing a large quantity of cancer cells*, which does not take the impact on the immune system and the closely related issue of survival rate into consideration. Since the dosage of antineoplastic drugs is determined in accordance with such a criterion, it is evident that the immunity will be wrecked during the course and the treatment itself may not aid in extending the remaining lifespan of the patient.

It is best to apply a balanced dosage to damage cancer cells and to preserve the immunity at the same time. However, the routine practice is to provide the maximum tolerated dose for the destruction of the greatest amount of cancer cells, where it leads to the breakdown of the immune system and holds back the attack against cancer cells. This is the chief shortcoming of the standard of care. During the past ten years, while the *five-year survival rate* for early cancer has been improved significantly by the standard of care, the same improvement has not been observed in patients diagnosed with advanced cancer that has been surviving after unsuccessful resection or relapsing post-operatively. In my opinion, the treatment response in advanced cancer is limited when the current standard of care is given.

When it comes to cancer treatment, spontaneously it is referred to as the standard of care in almost every hospital. If the patient is not equipped with any medical knowledge, he/she could only take the professional advice and accept the standard of care. Based on my observation, patients who would like to inquire about the usage of Opdivo® has increased since Professor Tasuku Honjo won the Nobel Prize in 2018.

Unquestionably, it is utterly shocking to be diagnosed as having cancer, and it may be a much easier way to rely on the professional suggestions rather than to search for the cure on one's own. Nevertheless, the continuous of the standard of care weakens the immune system and causes resistance to antineoplastic agents. Eventually, many patients who are struggling to survive find themselves left with nowhere to go, confronted by bad news that leads to the conclusion that "there is nothing we can do now" or "palliative care may be an option for your current condition."

By improving the immunity, we have been treating many desperate patients and prolonging the lifespan of stage 4 cancer patients who were unresponsive to the standard of care as well as pancreatic cancer patients with poor prognosis for an extension of 1, 3, or 5 years. In addition to the standard of care, our hospital provides other cancer treatments based on the concept of *immunity-focusing therapy*. Basically, our treatment protocol involves hyperthermia therapy, Opdivo®—the anticancer immunotherapy agent—and low-dose antineoplastic drugs. Many papers have suggested that when administered in a minimal amount, the immune system may be activated by the application of antineoplastic medicines. Recently, it has been shown that more than 90% of our patients have experienced a recovery with the addition of hydrogen. Besides medical practitioners, any person who has ever dug into cancer treatment may have an rough idea about how astounding this statistic is.

The Reason Why the Standard of Care Fails to Cure Terminal Cancer

The news that Professor Tasuku Honjo won the 2018 Nobel Prize was released like a giant bomb shaking the long-standing practice of cancer treatment. In fact, the news was deemed to declare that "terminal cancer can be cured by using Opdivo® to relieve the immunosuppression." That is to say, proper immune induction has the potential to cure end-stage cancer. However, the three major types of cancer treatment performed by the majority of hospitals not only wipe out cancer cells, but also destroy the immune system. There is no treatment given in consideration of the impact on the patients' immune system, and that is the reason why the standard of care has failed to treat terminal cancer.

Even though Opdivo® has been used in cancer centers recently, it has been applied simply as one of the antineoplastic drugs. It seems that many among the specialists in favor of antineoplastic treatments have not taken the immune issue into account. As a result, Opdivo® has been considered as just a single type of antineoplastic drugs, while it is best to be used as an immunotherapy agent. From my perspective, cancer is an illness caused by immune system dysfunction and therefore is best treated by an oncology specialist.

The Number of Six Hundred Thousand Cancer Refugees Continues to Grow

Public hospitals, such as medical centers and university hospitals, provide treatment in compliance with the national guideline. A large hospital is essentially an enterprise full of systems and hierarchies that are managed by different sources of authority, it would not be easy to offer treatments other than the standard of care. As the person in charge of an institution, I am unfettered to perform immune-based cancer treatment and different therapies aside from the standard of care. But then, from a managerial point of view, following the guideline to offer the standard of care secures a certain level of profit. To think as an executive, it would be a safer choice to perform the standard of care for the administrative stability of the hospital.

Additionally, it is not practical to provide self-paid medical services in hospitals adhering to the standard of care. The Japanese law specifically prohibits the concurrent provision of NHI-subsidized services and self-paid services, namely a mixed service. In any given day, in the event that the mixed service is provided by a single medical facility, the NHI subsidy will not be applicable for the patient receiving such services. The payment supposedly covered by the NHI will end up being converted into the actual expense of the patient, placing a substantial financial burden on them. In any way, the options for cancer treatment are limited.

Because of this, many doctors may only offer the standard of care that is applicable to the NHI and supported by the guideline, despite the variety of cancer treatments. Yet, antineoplastic drugs that destroy cancer cells and immune cells altogether may lose their potency gradually in the long term. Ultimately, doctors are forced to conclude that "there is nothing we can do now" or "the time to consider palliative care may have come." Patients become the so-called *cancer refugees* who are left helpless and lost to find the cure on their own. According to the estimation, the current number of cancer refugees in Japan has exceeded six hundred thousand people.

Basically, doctors in large hospitals do not discuss other available treatment options with the patient because the effectiveness of those methods has not yet been proven. In some cases, even when the patient asks about other possible choices, the doctor may dismiss the idea by answering, "oh, it doesn't work for you." At the end, patients would have to find out the solution for survival by themselves. In this modern age, many of them have attempted to search for the adequate treatment via internet comments or patient communications.

We have created a shelter for these desperate cancer refugees in our hospital. They have primarily come from all prefectures in Kyushu and many other places apart from Osaka, Nagoya, and Tokyo. Based on hydrogen therapy, we have performed many types of immunotherapies to help cancer patients who were once given up by their doctors regain health. We take pride in what we do, and we believe that our work is the source of our joy as medical practitioners.

One Specific Treatment to Save Cancer Refugees

Immune activation is most important for terminal cancer patients especially. It is crucial to realize there are many approaches to cancer treatment instead of just one. The induction of the leading role of the immunity—CD8 killer T cells—fails with hindrance to any step involved in the CIC. In other words, the induction failure can be caused by more than one factor. It is important to take advantage of personal immune indices for the prevention of such failure. Meanwhile, it is recommended to apply a combination of a few treatments correspondingly to find out the best way to boost the immunity. Immune enhancement is not only related to cancer treatment, but also to the alleviation of all forms of discomfort. The practice of immune improvement in our daily lives is beneficial to prevent cancer development, promote cancer recovery, and stay healthy after treatment.

Currently, *hyperthermia therapy* is one of the immunotherapies used in cancer treatment. Hyperthermia therapy is a method which employs an 8MHz high frequency wave to increase the central temperature of the lesion to 42°C or above, resulting in the selective death of cancer cells. In addition, the peripheral temperature of the lesion would reach a level of approximately 40°C , which maximizes the immune activity and particularly activates dendritic cells participated in Step 2 and Step 3 of the CIC. In the meantime, as the tumor vascularity improves with the increased temperature, Steps 4 and 5 of the CIC are facilitated by an increased number of immune cells arriving at the tumor site. Besides, an added bonus is that hyperthermia therapy is a treatment method applicable to the NHI subsidy.

The usage of low-dose antineoplastic drugs is another factor to consider. It has been suggested that the application of a standard dose destroys everything including immune cells, whereas a low dose equal to the amount of one third to one fourth of the standard dose activates the immune system. Medications applicable to the NHI subsidy and suitable for low-dose usage may include paclitaxel, gemcitabine, and cisplatin. Opdivo®, also known as nivolumab, is commonly used as an immune checkpoint inhibitor. It is effective in preventing cancer cells from putting up the defense mechanism of PD-L1 expression after being attacked by activated T cells. According to the current regulation, all cases requiring the usage of Opdivo® are categorized as self-paid services, except for lung cancer, stomach cancer, head and neck cancer, renal cancer, malignant lymphoma, and melanoma.

In my hospital, hydrogen has been monitored to enhance the efficacy of the above-mentioned treatments. While the details are discussed in the following chapters, so far it has been clearly shown that **hydrogen energizes killer T cells and promotes the efficacy of Opdivo®**. Given its high potency, hydrogen therapy has become one of the popular treatments among my patients, even though it is not eligible for the NHI subsidy.

In summary, cancer treatment does not just include antineoplastic drugs and radiation therapy. I believe part of the mission of a medical practitioner, after acquiring a thorough understanding of all the available treatment methods, is to consider the patients' medical and financial conditions and to advise the optimal treatment option for them.

Chapter 3

Immune Deficiency Is an Obstacle to the Success of Antineoplastic drugs and Radiotherapy

The Reason Why Current Treatment Options Aren't Working

Until now, the *standard of care*, consisting of surgical operations, antineoplastic drugs, and radiation therapy, has been recognized as the standard anticancer treatment and provided in accordance with guidelines established by relevant associations. While patients diagnosed with early cancer may be cured by receiving the standard of care, patients suffering from advanced cancer may or may not respond to such treatment and may fail in their attempts on *life extension*. Especially for terminal cancer patients, the standard of care is not the appropriate treatment for them.

As we have mentioned earlier, surgical procedures, antineoplastic drugs, and radiotherapy performed as the standard of care can cause devastating damage to the immune system while reducing the tumor size. Once immune dysfunction occurs, T cell deficiency sure follows. T cells become incompetent to identify and remove residual cancer cells in the body, which results in a condition that neglects and allows cancer proliferation. From a microscopic point of view, there is a considerable amount of remaining cancer cells even when the tumor mass is temporarily reduced or disappeared. Besides, it has been alleged that our bodies produce five thousand cancer cells each day. This will not cause a problem when the immune system is up and well. Yet when the immune system is down and weakened, cancer growth may become unstoppable.

By nature, the immune system is in charge of the identification, attack, and removal of foreign substances. Nonetheless, the administration of the standard of care inflicts severe damage on the immune system, disabling immune cells from killing cancer cells. As a result, the tumor expands once more and necessitates the re-administration of antineoplastic drugs or radiotherapy. Then again, following the second treatment, the tumor shrinks tentatively, but the immune system is struck more fiercely. This leads to another episode of cancer reproduction and relapse where antineoplastic drugs and radiotherapy become futile. A recent report discussing the association of antineoplastic drug resistance with immune inhibitory molecules has also suggested that the immune condition is closely related to treatment failure of antineoplastic agents.

Under the circumstances, it is almost certain that doctors are at their wits' end and may have to give up on their patients. In Japan, approximately six hundred thousand people yearning to survive have parted with the medical system, becoming desperate cancer refugees, wandering and lost in their way. In a survey conducted in the University of Tokyo Hospital by a newspaper called "Chunichi Shimbun," a question about "how would you like to face your death?" received the answer that "I wish to pass on after trying all available treatments" from 95% of the patients and 51% of the doctors. Perhaps this conceptual discrepancy between the role of patients and doctors is one of the contributing factors to cancer refugees.

The standard of care is, of course, effective to some patients and gives rise to high treatment success rates in patients with early cancer. However, it is not as equally effective in patients with terminal cancer. The treatment goal of the standard of care has been primarily focused on the *devastation of cancer cells,* rather than *prolongation of life expectancy*. But then, did you know what the effectiveness criterion of cancer treatment is? With regard to the standard of care, the treatment is considered *effective* when the size of a malignant tumor is reduced within 4 weeks. And it *remains effective* even if the tumor regrows and enlarges afterwards. In my opinion, it is unreasonable and unacceptable to incorporate treatments fulfilling such a lenient criterion as the standard of care.

The respective guidelines for surgical procedures, antineoplastic drugs, and radiotherapy distinctly indicate that *the treatment can only be provided via these routes*. This simply means *in the event that the treatment given according to the guidelines fails, there is no alternative for the patient.* Even if the tumor size is tentatively reduced by the use of antineoplastic agents, the tumor is going to regrow and enlarge in the case of immune deficiency. A well-functioning immune system is critical for sustainable tumor reduction and inhibition of cancer proliferation. Thus, T cells must be activated to increase the immunity and to attack cancer cells.

When we consider antineoplastic treatment of advanced cancer (unresectable or recurrent cancer), the proportion of patients showing a reduced tumor size is 30% at most, and this reduction can only be observed in the first and second treatment courses. The third and fourth treatment courses, referred to as the third and fourth schemes in the guidelines, seem *almost useless* from a doctor's perspective. It would be a miracle if the antineoplastic treatment works in the third or fourth courses. In principle, the more the treatment, the less effective it may be. Nevertheless, since no alternative treatment options can be offered other than the standard of care, even if knowing the third and fourth courses are doomed to failure, doctors would have to continue till the treatment is proven ineffective. Only until then can they admit that "we are finally up against the wall."

The dosage of antineoplastic drugs is determined by the guideline, which describes that "the maximum dose is calculated by taking the weight divided by the body surface area and should be equal to or no greater than X mg." This information is lapped up by many physicians without a doubt. While the provision of the maximum dose specified in the standard of care may decrease the tumor size occasionally, the immune system would also be wrecked to lower the inhibition of cancer proliferation immediately.

The importance of maintaining a strong immune system for the patient is noted by few doctors. Most practitioners have learned to concentrate on the elimination of cancer cells, giving no thoughts to the treatment impact on the immune system. Still, doctors who choose to comply with the current guidelines have constituted the majority. While some of them may have realized that the transient effect of antineoplastic treatment could neither cure the patients nor extend their lives, many have not made up their minds to change their treatment protocols because of the overall obstacles they have faced. In spite of that, it is my belief that a doctor should try to understand the struggle of patients, listen to their cries which convey their eagerness for survival, and provide the treatment with the aim of prolonging their lives till the end.

Even Cancer Experts Have No Idea about the Importance of Immunity

The normal function of the immune system is essential to the success of cancer treatment. I have once heard about doctors dismissing the inquiry about immunotherapies by replying, "well, that simply doesn't work." It is discouraging to know that although many professionals have attended immunology programs at medical school, some may find it uneasy to accept the relevant concepts. The word "antigen," which is referred to as the specific proteins existing in cancer cells, has only become well known until the 1990s, and the field of immunology has only started to develop since then. In a sense, doctors graduated anytime before that may have little knowledge of these areas unless they have continued the education by themselves.

Immunology is closely related to cancer treatment, and yet the treatment involved with Opdivo® has only been established after the year 2000. Opdivo® is an immune checkpoint inhibitor. To put it simply, Opdivo® works by removing the impediment to cancer destruction and resuming the attack of T cells against cancer cells. After Distinguished Professor Tasuku Honjo of the Kyoto University won the 2018 Nobel Prize for his research on Opdivo®, relevant courses may have become available at medical school. However, it seems that no courses have been set up at universities to discuss the role of immunology in cancer treatment.

The current cancer treatment is mainly based on the *standard of care*, which consists of operational procedures, antineoplastic drugs, and radiation therapy. Since these approaches are the treatment options offered by the majority of doctors, the patients' knowledge of other cancer therapies may be restricted. While killing cancer cells, the performance of the standard of care may cause damage to the immune system, and therefore many cases of relapse have been reported despite transient tumor reduction. It has been estimated that 90% of patients with stage 4 cancer who have only received the standard of care have died.

Nonetheless, various treatment approaches exist besides the standard of care. Among them, I have been studying and treating patients with *immunotherapies* which are effective in improving the immunity against cancer. And I have been trying to take the patient's condition into consideration when selecting and recommending the most adequate treatment method, which I believe would become the routine practice for the future cancer treatment.

The Cancer-Immunity Cycle Is the Key to Cancer Prevention

When it comes to cancer immunotherapy, it is important to understand the above-mentioned *cancer-immunity cycle (CIC)*. As an immuno-oncology specialist, I have seen many patients with stage 4 cancer experiencing tumor reduction or disappearance and maintaining stable conditions with the help of a proper functioning CIC. It has been said that the human body generates five thousand cancer cells in a day, and a normal CIC is the reason why some of us manage to stay healthy. This cycle also works properly in patients demonstrating tumor reduction or disappearance.

As described below, the CIC is a 7-step framework in which hindrance to any of the steps precludes its normal operation. The malfunction of the CIC is related to unregulated proliferation of cancer cells, cancer development, or recurrence. Thus, the top priority for cancer treatment of stage 4 patients is to maintain a well-functioning CIC to achieve immune enhancement.

The steps involved in the CIC

1. Cancer cell impairment by antineoplastic drugs or radiation therapy
2. Absorption of cancer cells damaged in Step 1 and expression of tumor markers by dendritic cells which are categorized as immune cells
3. T cell education and activation by dendritic cells for tumor marker identification
4. Transportation of activated T cells for tumor hunting
5. T cell infiltration to the tumor site.
6. T cell recognition of the tumor.
7. T cell attack on the tumor.

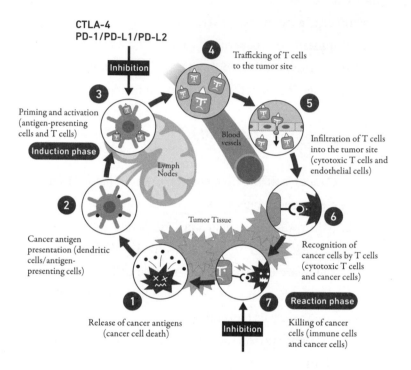

CTLA-4
PD-1/PD-L1/PD-L2

Inhibition

4 Trafficking of T cells to the tumor site

3 Priming and activation (antigen-presenting cells and T cells)

Induction phase

Blood vessels

5 Infiltration of T cells into the tumor site (cytotoxic T cells and endothelial cells)

Lymph Nodes

2 Cancer antigen presentation (dendritic cells/antigen-presenting cells)

Tumor Tissue

6 Recognition of cancer cells by T cells (cytotoxic T cells and cancer cells)

1 Release of cancer antigens (cancer cell death)

Inhibition

7 Killing of cancer cells (immune cells and cancer cells)

Reaction phase

Induction phase:	Antigen-presenting cells express cancer antigens to T cells (initial stage)
Reaction phase:	T cells are activated to identify cancer antigens and elicit the immune response (action stage)

To Build a Robust Body with Your Immunity Is of the Utmost Importance

90% of my patients have suffered from stage 4 cancer. With regard to: With regard to patients who have been unresponsive to antineoplastic drugs in the standard of care, a combination of immunotherapies has been given in our hospital to deliver the optimal treatment. Indeed, we have managed to prolong the remaining lifespan for a couple of years in patients expected with three months left only.

I have believed in the absolute importance of immune enhancement during cancer treatment. However, there have been no available methods to assess the baseline immunity and the actual level of immune improvement achieved by the performance of immunotherapies. It is not an easy task to provide evidence or scientific basis for these treatments, and this may be one of the factors contributing to the rejection of immunotherapies by many practitioners.

Having said that, we have created a system in our hospital to measure the immune level using venous blood samples. The assay is conducted by SRL, Inc., one of the best laboratory service companies in Japan. This system examines the immune condition of the patient to assist in the selection of the possibly optimal treatment.

According to the data acquired from this system, it is intriguing to note that the number of people who have a stronger immune system is essentially equal to those with a weaker immune system. And it may be concluded that, based on a percentage of 50% for each group, roughly half of the Japanese population are predisposed to cancer because of low immunity. These data are consistent with the information provided by the Ministry of Health, Labor and Welfare of Japan, which indicated that one in every two Japanese may be diagnosed with cancer throughout one's lifetime. At present, cancer patients are required to receive such an examination. Yet by early screening with this test, expansion of cancer prevention may be possible.

Chapter 4

Curing End-Stage Cancer Patients With Hydrogen

How Can Hydrogen Help to Enhance Immunity?

There are two major effects of hydrogen on cancer treatment: selective removal of the bad reactive oxygen species (ROS) and mitochondrial activation. Firstly, let's begin with explaining the mechanism of the former. While we breathe in oxygen, the by-product of oxygen consumption is called ROS. There are four types of ROS, including superoxide anion (or superoxide), hydrogen peroxide, singlet oxygen, and hydroxyl free radical (or hydroxyl radical). Superoxide anion, hydrogen peroxide, and singlet oxygen are categorized as the good ROS which helps to activate the immune system, whereas hydroxyl free radicals are addressed as the bad ROS that may decrease the immunity.

Among them, hydroxyl free radicals are harmful to the human body. The bad ROS promotes oxidation processes which give rise to skin speckles and dullness as well as low energy, and may become the cause of various diseases, such as cancer, diabetes, pneumonia, myocardial infarction, and Alzheimer's disease. The main mechanism of action, i.e. the interaction with the human body, of hydroxyl free radicals is to damage blood vessels and

DNA. In particular, the bad ROS impairs mitochondrial DNA, restrains mitochondrial energy production, and results in declining cellular function, bringing significant damage to immune cells specifically.

Selectively, hydrogen removes the bad ROS without affecting the good ones and thus plays an important role in immune enhancement. This is one of the key features of hydrogen that matter the most. Many patients have believed that taking dietary antioxidative supplements is the most effective way to inhibit oxidation processes and the bad ROS. However, it has been reported in a recent study that taking dietary antioxidative supplements does not prevent aging-related diseases and may instead raise the risk of mortality.

In detail, the study result suggests that intake of popular dietary supplements containing vitamin E and dietary products containing beta-carotene may lead to an increased mortality rate of 4% and 7% compared to placebo, respectively. An increased risk of lung cancer has also been reported. Presumably, dietary antioxidative supplements suppress the level of the bad and good ROS altogether. On the other hand, selective removal of the bad ROS by hydrogen is highly contributable to immunotherapies, which can be deemed as a significant breakthrough in cancer treatment.

What Exactly Is Hydrogen?

Hydrogen is remembered by many of us as the first element listed in the periodic table with an atomic number of 1. Hydrogen is constituted by one electron and one proton. It is known to be the lightest element and the substance formed at the beginning of the universe.

The universe was created 15 billion years ago. After 3 hundred thousand years, electrons and protons gathered to form the first element—hydrogen. Carbon, nitrogen, and iron were created during subsequent fusion reactions. At the present time, hydrogen is accounted for 90% of the elements constituting the universe. It is estimated that prior to the emergence of Homo sapiens 3 billion years ago, hydrogen has long existed on Earth.

As we all know, hydrogen is an odorless and tasteless gas at room temperature with very high diffusivity. The use of hydrogen bomb may give an impression of a sense of danger, while in actual, hydrogen can only be burned when its concentration reaches above 4%. Besides, since the hydrogen molecules are diffused all over under normal condition, it is almost impossible for hydrogen to gather and explode.

The existence of hydrogen is natural to the universe. In 1766, British chemist and physicist Henry Cavendish combined metallic plates and strong acids to discover the "inflammable air (which is known as hydrogen today)" for the first time. In 1783, French scholar Antoine Lavoisier coined the name "hydrogen."

Based on the description of the International Atomic Energy Agency (IAEA), hydrogen is the third most abundant element (10%) found in the body, following oxygen (61%) and carbon (23%). Apart from water, hydrogen is the composition of proteins, nuclear acids, and lipids of the human body, which makes it indispensable to our daily lives. Hydrogen has been surrounding us ever since mankind was first seen on Earth. I believe hydrogen can be potentially beneficial to significant improvement of the human immunity.

Lift the Immunosuppression to Achieve Successful Treatment Outcome

Former immunotherapies involved the use of the fungus family of Polyporaceae (ganoderma), specific substance Maruyama, and Hasumi vaccine. Although they could be *potentially helpful*, the efficacy of these therapies could not be validated. In addition, the immune cell therapy utilizing the patient's own lymphocytes has not shown supportive evidence for its effectiveness. Perhaps these similar events helped shape the stereotype of *ineffective immunotherapies* among doctors complying with the standard of care.

However, the treatment response of *hydrogen immunotherapy* (the combination of previous immunotherapies and hydrogen) is fairly obvious. From the evidence or scientific basis constructed by me through the collection of over 400 cases in March 2019, it can be noted, as one of the key features of **hydrogen immunotherapy, that hydrogen may help to enable mitochondrial activation and lift the immunosuppression.**

So far, as we have discussed the idea of cancer inhibition via immune activation, the critical point has been lying in the activation of the human immunity in every possible way. Yet, the human body may simultaneously initiate immune activation and suppression. On the one hand, our physical health is left unguarded when the immune system fails to maintain its normal function. On the other hand, an overactive immune system may turn around and attack ourselves. Thus, it is necessary for our bodies to initiate the *immunosuppression* spontaneously.

During the course of cancer treatment, the immune system becomes activated because of the presence of cancer antigens/tumor markers. This would bring about an equal or even stronger level of immunosuppression, counteracting and holding back the immune attack against cancer cells. As a result, the immunosuppression must be lifted to maintain the normal function of the immune system and resume cancer elimination. Opdivo® is a potent agent designed to relieve the immunosuppression, though it seems to cause side effects including interstitial pneumonia and diabetes. The cytoplasmic process involved in Opdivo® mechanism of immunosuppression relief is described as follows.

Immunosuppression relieved by Opdivo®

1. T cells become activated to attack cancer cells, i.e. immune activation.

2. T cells produce immunosuppressive molecules—PD-1—to prevent overactivation and self-attack, i.e. immune suppression.

3. Opdivo® combines with PD-1 to inactivate the immunosuppression, i.e. immune activation.

*Opdivo® lifts the immunosuppression by combining with PD-1 on T cells, whereas hydrogen prevents immune suppression via promoting mitochondrial activation and prohibiting PD-1 generation.

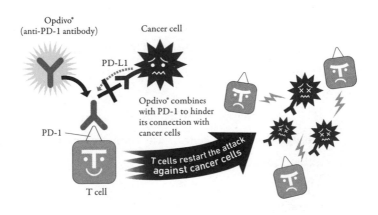

Action of the *immune checkpoint inhibitor*——Opdivo®
Opdivo® combines with PD-1 on T cells to block its connection with cancer cells so as to remove the obstacle to the immune response and resume T cell activation.

Compared to Opdivo®, hyperthermia therapy applied as part of immunotherapy and low-dose antineoplastic drugs may help to relieve the immunosuppression to a lesser degree without producing side effects. Similarly, hydrogen may be used to lift the *immunosuppression* too. Unlike Opdivo®, hydrogen does not combine with PD-1 on T cells to remove the immune suppression. Instead, hydrogen acts by blocking PD-1 generation to prevent the launch of immunosuppression in the first place.

Immunosuppression prohibited by hydrogen

1. Especially in patients with advanced cancer, T cells exhausted during a constant battle against cancer cells are called fatigued T cells. These T cells are prone to express PD-1 due to mitochondrial dysfunction.
2. **Hydrogen promotes mitochondrial activation in fatigued T cells to reactivate them for cancer cell destruction.**

Yet, consideration must be given that there are at least two types of T cells found with PD-1 expression, including *fatigued T cells* and T cells with normal mitochondrial function that are called *suppressor T cells*. Suppressor T cells are *activated T cells* capable of attacking cancer cells. And as part of the above-mentioned immune control mechanism, suppressor T cells may express PD-1 molecules to inhibit the immune function and prevent overactivation. In other words, the normal mitochondrial function of *suppressor T cells* is the key factor that brings Opdivo® into play.

The other type of T cells presenting with PD-1 is *fatigued T cells* which have become exhausted during a long battle against cancer cells. One of the major characteristics of fatigued T cells is the inability to remove cancer cells because of mitochondrial dysfunction. Therefore, Opdivo® is not useful in helping fatigued T cells despite the fact that PD-1 presentation can be found on these T cells. Even though Opdivo® binds with PD-1 to block the channel of immunosuppression,fatigued T cells may remain disabled due to mitochondrial malfunctioning. This may partially explain why Opdivo® only works in 20% to 30% of cancer patients.

While Opdivo® lifts the immunosuppression through the combination with PD-1, hydrogen reduces PD-1 expression by promoting mitochondrial activation to energize T cells. That is, hydrogen increases our innate immunity without affecting our body function. Although the *end result* of counteracting immunosuppression induced by PD-1 molecules is the same, it is important to understand the mechanism of action is completely different between hydrogen and Opdivo®. The immunosuppression relief achieved by hydrogen is not artificial and follows natural processes so that no side effects will be caused. **The *immunosuppression* must be relieved to allow the immune system to launch fierce attack against cancer cells, which is especially important for end-stage cancer patients.**

In general, PD-1-expressing T cells found in advanced or terminal cancer patients are mostly *fatigued T cells* suffering from mitochondrial dysfunction. Therefore, as we have just discussed, Opdivo® is not an effective option under such condition, and the only available method to reactivate fatigued T cells and achieve immune activation is hydrogen application. Exhibiting the same effect as Opdivo®, hydrogen is a potentially promising treatment approach that does not lead to side effects in advanced or terminal cancer patients who were unresponsive to Opdivo®.

Hydrogen Increases Opdivo® Response Rate by 40%

It has been clear that *hydrogen immunotherapy* which combines hydrogen and previous immunotherapies is beneficial to reorganize the process of the cancer-immunity cycle (CIC) (see Chapter 1, p.46). For stage 4 cancer patients, hydrogen application helps to increase the response rate of Opdivo® from 20%-30% to 60%-70%. The CIC is a series of steps involved with the induction of *recognition and destruction of cancer cells by T cells.* Generally, there are three types of T cells, including the energetic *killer T cells*, *suppressor T cells* with PD-1 presentation and normal mitochondrial function, as well as *fatigued T cells* suffering from mitochondrial dysfunction.

In order to prevent an overactive immune system, the human body initiates the immunosuppression by expressing PD-1 molecules on activated T cells to transform them into suppressor T cells. The mechanism of Opdivo® is to remove the obstacle of T cell-mediated immunosuppression by combining with PD-1. However, the immunosuppressive effect may not be relieved through the binding of Opdivo® and PD-1 molecules on fatigued T cells. To deal with this problem, the fundamental cause of *fatigued T cells*—mitochondrial dysfunction—must be solved first.

Regarding the solution, hydrogen is a mighty tool

to achieve mitochondrial activation in *fatigued T cells* and to further convert them back into *activated T cells*. But the conversion may not be 100%, some of them may turn into *suppressor T cells* with PD-1 expression and improved mitochondrial function. Patients receiving Opdivo® treatment are mostly diagnosed with stage 4 cancer, and the majority of T cells found in these patients is comprised of *fatigued T cells*. As a result, the response rate of Opdivo® is often limited to 20%-30%, since the immunosuppressive effect may not be easily lifted through the combination of Opdivo® and PD-1 molecules on fatigued T cells.

However, the response rate may be increased up to 60%-70% with the addition of hydrogen inhalation prior to the administration of Opdivo®. This is because hydrogen achieves mitochondrial activation in *fatigued T cells* and turns them into *activated T cells* or *suppressor T cells* which are sensitive to the action of Opdivo®. Opdivo® monotherapy demonstrates positive outcome on *suppressor T cells*, while it exerts no effect on *fatigued T cells*. On the other hand, it is generally believed that hydrogen is effective in activating *fatigued T cells* and converting the greater part of them into activated T cells that would attack cancer cells instantly without the help of Opdivo®.

It is assumed that while hydrogen transforms most of T cells into *activated T cells*, a small number of *suppressor T cells* remains and must be tackled by the use of Opdivo®. Thus, it is significant to apply the combination of hydrogen and a minimum amount of Opdivo® to achieve sufficient treatment effect. Likewise, **it is typically thought that hydrogen is effective for advanced and end-stage patients who are found with myriads of *fatigued T cells*, whereas Opdivo® is futile for these patients except in combination with hydrogen.**

For patients suffering from advanced or terminal cancer and showing no response to Opdivo®, hydrogen therapy is a novel promising approach to offer similar efficacy to Opdivo® without causing any side effects. In other words, hydrogen application for cancer treatment is equal to a *new weapon* for the battle of life prolongation.

Hydrogen Inhalation Causes No Pain and Suffering

Hydrogen therapy results in neither side effects of medication nor adverse reactions from overconsumption. Hydrogen is the smallest molecule among all available substances. Although the body filters out undesired materials naturally, it is speculated that there may have been residual hydrogen deep in the lungs.

It was reported that 69 ppm of exhaled hydrogen was measured at 8 AM subsequent to hydrogen inhalation at 1 AM on the same day. Under normal condition, the amount of hydrogen measured in exhaled air is 7-8 ppm. After comparison, it is obvious that a significant amount of hydrogen can be accumulated within the body. It is my belief that the maintenance of high levels of hydrogen may help remove the bad ROS accountable for various diseases and keep a high level of immunity.

In our hospital, hydrogen immunotherapy performed for terminal cancer patients requires the use of a machine for hydrogen supply equal to or greater than 1200 ml per minute. The treatment protocol stipulates at least 3 hours of hydrogen inhalation per day. Most patients would choose to divide the course into one hour each in the morning, noon, and evening. While receiving hydrogen inhalation, patients are allowed to sleep, read, watch TV, or basically do anything that helps them relax. Yet to enhance treatment effect, my personal recommendation is to meditate.

It is easy to go into a meditative state after receiving hydrogen inhalation. But the generation of theta wave is promoted if you consciously create an environment suitable for meditation during hydrogen inhalation. The frequency of theta wave ranges from 4 to 7 Hz, which occurs while you enter a state between sleep and awakening. In this phase, you may experience a sudden inspiration or memory improvement, and this is the best condition for the natural healing power to come into play. As a result, the treatment effect of hydrogen inhalation is greatly increased when the patient lies still and closes the eyes. It is important to relax and keep a steady mind in the long journey against cancer, and so it may be helpful to calm down like this for a few hours every day.

Additionally, there is a timer on the hydrogen equipment to assign the course duration or to operate in the continuous mode. Hydrogen molecules are tiny substances which can be filtered out by the human body. Thus, it is needless to worry about adverse reactions arisen from overconsumption. Hydrogen inhibits the growth of cancer cells and improves the immunity through natural processes without causing side effects. In contrast, medication is certainly accompanied by side effects because it is an artificial method that forces the manifestation of treatment effect. Also, medication surely causes impairment to certain body parts, which exhibits in the form of side effects. Hydrogen therapy is irrelevant to these problems. Instead, it is a treatment approach that benefits the body and induces the natural healing power smoothly.

One of the severe side effects resulted from antineoplastic drugs or radiation therapy in the standard of care is the breakdown of the immune system. Other symptoms, including nausea, anemia, tiredness, and hair loss, have been seen in many patients and have affected their daily lives. When it comes to cancer treatment, there is always a strong impression of severe side effects. It is my intention to inform the public about treatment like hydrogen therapy, which helps to increase our innate healing power and to promote healthy recovery.

Don't Be Afraid to Know Your Remaining Lifespan. Hydrogen Is Your Helper for Cancer Elimination

Many stage 4 patients have experienced tumor reduction or disappearance with continuous hydrogen immunotherapy. As introduced in the foreword (p.25),

Ms. K · H is one of the most remarkable examples. Ms. K · H had lymph node metastasis and was presented with a large mass under her jaw, and so she was admitted to our hospital immediately. However, after receiving hydrogen immunotherapy, the mass was gone completely within two weeks and Ms. K · H was discharged in good condition. Subsequently, the value of her tumor marker had decreased significantly.

Even though hydrogen is highly beneficial, it is extremely rare to observe symptom improvement within such a short time. For most patients, tumor reduction may start to occur after 2 to 3 months of hydrogen immunotherapy. That is the time it takes for T cells to be activated by hydrogen and begin attacking cancer cells. Yet, the treatment should be continued for some time in spite of tumor reduction or disappearance. Residual cancer cells are often detected in cancer that seems vanished. And even if the cancer does disappear, there are 5 thousand cancer cells produced in our bodies every day. A decreased level of immunity resulted from treatment termination increases the risk of cancer regrowth. Remember, the immune power that defeats the cancer is derived from the treatment, rather than the original immunity of the patient.

Hence, caution is required even when cancer

disappears. While receiving cancer treatment, it is necessary to integrate treatments designed for immune enhancement so as to maintain high immunity and reduce the tumor size until the innate immunity is strong enough to identify and eliminate cancer cells. Alternatively, treatment should be continued to achieve coexistence with cancer. People who were told to "have only 3 months left" have undergone these treatments in our hospital and prolonged their own lives for a couple of years. During this extension, they have managed to arrange things, enjoy the time spent with their family, visit the people they wish to see...and they have been content with every single day of living. In order to fulfill the intense eagerness of stage 4 patients to *fight until the end*, I am dedicated to providing the most adequate treatment method for them.

Hydrogen Activates Mitochondria to Boost Your Immunity!

One of the main characteristics of hydrogen immunotherapy is mitochondrial activation achieved by hydrogen. Mitochondria are cellular organelles responsible for a vital task that is linked to our own survival—intracellular energy supply. Mitochondria can also be found in T cells, the indispensable actor in immunotherapy.

T cells are important to the detection and destruction of cancer cells, while they may become impaired and fatigued because of antineoplastic drugs or radiotherapy. Mitochondrial activation achieved by hydrogen inhalation helps fatigued T cells to recover and restart the attack against cancer cells, leading to an increased immune response.

What Are Mitochondria?

Humans need energy to think, work, and talk, and the structure designed for energy production is called a mitochondrion. Mitochondria extract energy from the food we consume and transform it into the form that is usable by our bodies—ATP (adenosine triphosphate). ATP consumption is required for body movement and metabolism. Besides mankind, mitochondria are presented in every cell of all organisms including animals, plants, and fungi.

As we age, a decline in mitochondrial function occurs

because of the change of our physical condition or the accumulation of the bad ROS resulted from dietary and lifestyle factors. It has been reported that the bad ROS affects mitochondrial DNA and leads to mitochondrial dysfunction. In that case, mitochondria remain inactive even if antineoplastic drugs or radiotherapy is provided.

Moreover, mitochondria can also be found in T cells which are highly related to the immunity. A reduction in mitochondrial function results in T cell deficiency, which hinders T cells from attacking cancer cells and leads to unregulated cancer proliferation. To prevent this, it is important to achieve mitochondrial activation in our daily lives so as to resuscitate fatigued T cells for cancer inhibition and tumor reduction. For cancer patients, mitochondrial activation or immune enhancement is an essential element of cancer treatment.

Mitochondria Are the Energy Factory of the Human Body

Mitochondria play a vital role in immune activation and are strongly associated with hydrogen immunotherapy. So how do they work inside us? Well, there are two systems that produce energy for our bodies, namely the glycolytic system and the mitochondrial energy generating system (MEGS). These systems produce the basic form of energy—ATP—by distinct mechanisms.

Under low body temperature, the glycolytic system generates energy within the cytoplasm in the absence of oxygen. Cells undergoing repeated divisions, including

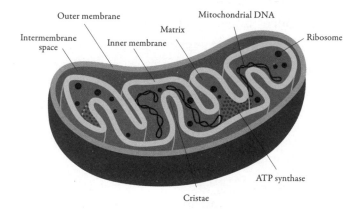

Mitochondria for energy production

Among the 4 trillion cells comprising the human body, each cell is presented with hundreds to thousands of mitochondria. Mitochondria are known to decompose nutrients and produce energy in the form of ATP (adenosine triphosphate).

regenerated epithelial tissue, bone marrow cells, cancer cells, skeletal muscles (white muscles), and sperms, rely on energy supply of the glycolytic system. Just like the energy required for sprinting, the energy provided by the glycolytic system is dedicated to instant muscular power.

In contrast, the MEGS uses oxygen to produce energy steadily within mitochondria under high body temperature. The efficiency of the MEGS is 16 times higher than the glycolytic system. Brain nerve cells (neurons), skeletal muscles (red muscles), cardiac muscles, and oocytes are dependent on energy produced by the MEGS. The usage of oxygen for energy production also results in fat burning. The energy provided by the MEGS is linked to aerobic exercise like walking.

In terms of the efficiency, the 16-time output production of the MEGS definitely prevails. That is, energy generated by the MEGS is delivered more efficiently and utilized in health promotion and maintenance. Additionally, continuous oxygen consumption of the MEGS is accompanied by ROS production. Among the four types of ROS derived, the bad ROS may become the cause of many illnesses, such as aging, cancer, and lifestyle diseases. And one of the major effects of hydrogen is to selectively remove the bad ROS to prevent subsequent oxidative reactions and to improve the functioning of ATP-generating mitochondria.

Fasting and exercise are closely related to our health. It has been proposed that the mechanism behind this involves sirtuin genes (also known as longevity genes) and ultimately achieves mitochondrial activation. While many of us may have learned that fasting and exercise are good to our health, it has become increasingly clear that things described to be *health promoting* are indeed in relation to mitochondrial activation. Once activated, sirtuin genes increase the mitochondrial energy production and facilitate cellular renewal by removing undesired proteins as well as aged mitochondria. Similar to mechanical renewal of an energy factory, cellular revitalization leads to immune enhancement and health improvement.

Fasting Increases Mitochondrial Activity

Mitochondria can be activated by exercise or fasting. In other words, physical stress is one of the factors that prompt energy production and thus promote mitochondrial activation. Fasting condition stimulates sirtuin genes (longevity genes) to activate PGC-1α molecules and to further produce and activate mitochondria. Consequently, T cells are activated to strengthen the immunity.

It is recommended to consult a healthcare professional prior to fasting in order to avoid unnecessary physical burdens and to prevent undesirable outcome resulted from the wrong practice. However, hydrogen inhalation activates PGC-1αmolecules through a similar mechanism, which may serve as a convenient alternative to fasting.

Hydrogen Improves Mitochondrial Function

Mitochondria account for 10% of the body weight, which is equal to a total of 6 kg in a person weighing 60 kg. In every single cell exist 1 hundred to 3 thousand mitochondria, so imagine how remarkable the number can be in a body consisting of 4 trillion cells. Indeed, it is possible to lengthen the healthy life expectancy through activation of such a huge amount of mitochondria.

However, it is difficult to keep mitochondrial DNA unharmed from our daily lives. Hydroxyl free radicals, the bad ROS produced along with breathing, lead to a decline in mitochondrial function, which decreases energy production for the body and results in low immunity. This condition may give rise to many types of disorders, such as skin speckles, wrinkles, arteriosclerosis, diabetes, dementia, and cancer.

In addition, PD-1 expression on T cells is increased in cancer patients. Among the population of healthy adults, however, the level of PD-1 presentation on T cells varies. In healthy people, T cells expressing PD-1 molecules are weakened, possibly due to mitochondrial dysfunction. From this perspective, people who have decreased mitochondrial function (increased PD-1 expression on T cells, equal to fatigued T cells found in cancer patients) are at a higher risk of developing cancer, pneumonia, or dementia.

In that case, hydrogen inhalation may help to suppress PD-1 presentation on T cells by removing the bad ROS and promoting mitochondrial activation, which may further prevent cancer, pneumonia, and dementia. Through the clearance of the bad ROS and the activation of PGC-1αmolecules, hydrogen inhalation is beneficial to significant improvement of mitochondrial function. Moreover, since mitochondrial quality is closely related to our health, it might be used as an adequate instrument in the future for prediction of disease development, life expectancy, and degenerative problems.

Mitochondria Quality, Good or Bad

Currently, there is a lack of a simple method to measure mitochondrial function. Yet, it has been suggested that the proportion of fatigued T cells in peripheral blood is highly associated with the prognosis of cancer patients. This has raised a question as to whether it also reflects mitochondrial function in T cells. And the answer to that question can be easily revealed by performing a routine blood test.

Such a test is significant in the battle against cancer. Nevertheless, examination of mitochondrial function for healthy people could help us take control of our own health and to prevent various diseases, including cancer, diabetes, stroke, and dementia. Based on the measurement of mitochondrial function, the healthy population can be categorized into people with better mitochondrial function and people with poorer mitochondrial function. This categorization is potentially useful in indicating disease development or even disclosing *pre-disease* condition to achieve *the visualization of prevention.*

Besides, it is generally believed that mitochondrial function is associated with telomere length. Located at the ends of chromosomes, the telomere shortens during each cell division as we grow old. The curtailed telomere drives cells towards the aging process instead of reproduction. It has been documented in the literature that mitochondrial dysfunction may lead to telomere shortening. In 2011, a research paper published in the journal *Nature* also suggested that the human lifespan is closely correlated with mitochondria.

Hydrogen inhalation removes the bad ROS, promotes metabolism, and improves mitochondrial function. It helps to ensure the wellness throughout the body, especially for the genes and vessels. Apart from cancer treatment, hydrogen elicits favorable changes in the body that lengthen the healthy life expectancy.

Chapter 5

Simple Habits to Boost Your Immunity

7 Ingredients to Improve Mitochondrial Health

By treating terminal cancer patients, we have disclosed the effectiveness of hydrogen and learned the important action of hydrogen—to achieve immune enhancement via mitochondrial activation. This discovery clearly indicates the fact that mitochondrial activation is indispensable to immune activation.

Fatigued T cells with PD-1 presentation can be found in different proportions across healthy people. As age increases, people who possess a greater amount of *fatigued T cells* increase. These people are at a higher risk of having geriatric pneumonia, cancer, dementia, etc., and are classified as the high-risk group.

However, hydrogen application is useful in mitochondrial activation and the reduction of *fatigued T cells* with PD-1 presentation. Through immune activation, hydrogen helps to prevent infection, cancer, dementia, and so on. **Hydrogen is not only effective in cancer treatment. In fact, just like any habits that promote mitochondrial activation, hydrogen is favorable for immune activation and is even beneficial to achieve healthy longevity.**

Apart from cancer patients, mitochondrial activation is a pragmatic approach to increase energy and improve health for everyone. If you wish to live in healthy longevity, it never hurts to build some habits that help to activate your mitochondria and increase your immunity. For instance, mitochondrial activation can be achieved by carefully selecting ingredients for your every meal. Coenzyme Q10 (CoQ10) is one of the enzymes located on the mitochondrial respiratory chain (intracellular enzymes associated with respiration). Responsible for delivering electrons from complexes I and II to complex III, CoQ10 plays an important role in mitochondrial energy production.

There are two types of CoQ10, the oxidized form and the reduced form. After ingestion, *the oxidized form* is required to be converted into the reduced form, whereas factors like aging, illness, and stress reduce this conversion rate. On the other hand, the structure of *the reduced form* is similar to CoQ10 generated in the body and therefore brings about immediate effects to support energy production. Consequently, it is important to ensure intake of *the reduced form* of CoQ10.

The ingredients listed below contain a relatively large amount of the reduced form of CoQ10. While the recommended dietary allowance of CoQ10 is 100 mg per day, no severe adverse reactions were shown up to the maximum intake of 300 mg per day in a study investigating the effect of 4-week consumption of CoQ10 in healthy Japanese participants.[†] Having said that, it is necessary to include plenty of vegetables and sufficient water in your diet to maintain nutritional balance for the optimal intake of the reduced form of CoQ10.

[†] Hosoe, et al. *Regulatory Toxicology and Pharmacology*, vol.47, 19-28, 2008

Ingredients rich in the reduced form of CoQ10

1. Wild pork: 140-200 ug/g
2. Ezo deer meat: 100-130 ug/g
3. Chicken heart: 84.8 ug/g
4. Beef liver: 40.1 ug/g
5. Pork shoulder: 25.41 ug/g
6. Amberjack: 20.9 ug/g
7. Soybean oil: 33.3 ug/g

Maximize Your Mitochondria with Aerobic Exercise

Adequate exercise is critical to healthy aging and to the increase of mitochondrial density. This section introduces a few types of exercise that help to increase mitochondrial numbers. Firstly, let's start from a quick briefing on a branch of the muscular system. Muscles that are used to voluntarily control movements of the trunk and extremities are called *skeletal muscles*. Skeletal muscles are mainly composed of *fast-twitch myofibers (fast muscles)* and *slow-twitch myofibers (slow muscles)*.

Fast muscles perform rapid contractions to exert great strength in a short time. In terms of land exercise, fast muscles are required for sprints. While these muscles are strong and powerful, they get exhausted easily due to a lack of muscular endurance. Fast muscles are also known as *white muscles* because they appear bright and pale. In contrast, slow muscles are so named since they contract at a slower speed. They are not a good candidate for intense bursts of energy but an outstanding source for long-lasting strength. These muscles are required for marathons as they are not easily tired. Slow muscles are also known as *red muscles* because of their reddish appearance.

Training for *slow muscles (red muscles)* assists in increasing mitochondrial density because the amount of mitochondria contained in slow-twitch myofibers is three times as much as in fast-twitch myofibers. Oxygen is the primary source of energy production in slow muscles. Thus, aerobic exercise, such as running, swimming, walking, and cycling, is more effective in training slow muscles.

Whilst low-intensity exercise raises mitochondrial density in slow muscles, a higher level of intensity maximizes the mitochondrial content in slow muscles and induces mitochondrial multiplication in fast muscles. Even though exercise increases mitochondrial level, discontinuation of exercise results in a gradual decrease in mitochondrial density. Hence, regular exercise is a much better choice compared to sporadically rigorous training. So, how would you like to perform some of the recommended aerobic exercises?

40°C Warm Water Baths and High-Quality Sleep Revitalize the Body

Hyperthermia therapy is one of the immunotherapies implemented in my hospital. Heated by a specialized device, cancer cells are killed when the central temperature of the lesion reaches 42℃- 43℃. At this point, the peripheral temperature is maintained at 40℃, a degree that is most effective in achieving immune activation. Therefore, taking a warm bath in 40 ℃ water helps to elevate your immune response. Instead of showering, my advice is to immerse your whole body below shoulders into warm water and relax yourself until you have some perspiration. This could also help to relieve your daily stress.

The autonomic nervous system comprises the sympathetic and parasympathetic nervous systems. The sympathetic nervous system prevails while we are working or doing house chores during the day, whereas the parasympathetic nervous system dominates when we feel relaxed and sleepy. This is what happens normally. In recent days, however, many people have experienced sympathetic dominance resulted from excessive stress and found themselves having trouble falling asleep.

Lack of high-quality sleep is one of the causes of immune deficiency. Thus, it is important to keep the parasympathetic nervous system in charge at night in order to have a sound sleep. Taking a warm bath to prepare for a good night of sleep may be a good idea. Yet, the high heat of a sauna could potentially activate the sympathetic nervous system. By contrast, a 40°C warm water bath is a better option for relaxation and immune enhancement. Moreover, water temperature of 38°C-40°C is most suitable for improving the quality of sleep. From shoulders to toes, immersing in such warm water for 10-15 minutes increases the body temperature as well as the metabolic and immune function. Meanwhile, the circulation is improved by water pressure while the body is supported by the buoyant force to ease muscle tension.

Furthermore, it is recommended to finish the bath 1 to 2 hours before bedtime in order to improve the quality of sleep. Sleepiness naturally occurs when the *core body temperature* drops. So the best timing to go to bed is 1 to 2 hours after the bath, when the core temperature starts to decrease. Although it is best to have 7 hours of sleep, sleep duration varies between individuals. Hormonal secretion and fatigue recovery reach the peak level during 10 PM to 2 AM and therefore it is important to sleep during this period to increase the quality of sleep.

In summer, many people may choose to sleep in an air-conditioned room. Please be aware that the coolness generated by the air conditioner lowers our body temperature slowly and decreases blood circulation as well as lymphatic and immune function. Cold stimulation like cooling the body momentarily by water spray, for example, activates mitochondria, whereas chronic coolness caused by the air conditioner reduces the immune response. So please bear this in mind and remember to set the timer.

Create Your Own Stress-Relief Strategies

Every one of us experiences stress more or less, as long as we are alive. A moderate level of stress is good to our physical and mental health, yet immense chronic stress is extremely harmful to the immunity.

Medical history is information required for the collection of previous medical conditions, background history, and family history during diagnosis of new patients. During the inquiry, many patients have admitted encountering enormous stress a couple of years prior to the onset. It is often said among doctors that many patients had lived a passive life and faced excessive stress for 4 or 5 years before they were diagnosed with cancer. Traumatic events, such as divorce, loss of a loved one, and unemployment, are major incidents that lead to instant decrease of immune function and cancer development. A severe level of mental stress is highly likely to impact the immunity.

While explaining the treatment protocol, I always ask my patients to *think about what makes you really happy*. But many reply that "I can't think about anything in particular" or "I am not particularly interested in anything." Stress-relieving strategies are crucial to an increased level of the immunity. Creating your own way of stress relief is vital to healthy aging. Please take your time to think about what actually makes you preoccupied and joyful, while it gives you a sense of achievement when it's done. Having something like this, even just one thing, helps to keep your immune system working properly at an advanced age.

Promote Bowel Health with Japanese Fermented Foods

The human intestine is home to more than one thousand types of bacteria, some of which can affect the immune system. In fact, a higher proportion of the bacterial species Ruminococcus Luminox and Faecalibacterium has been reported in patients responsive to Opdivo®, while a higher proportion of bacterioides has been observed in patients non-responsive to Opdivo®. The *intestinal flora* is a system containing a large number of intestinal bacteria which appear like "flower fields" under the microscope. Generally, intestinal bacteria can be categorized into the good, the bad, and the neutral bacteria.

Three types of intestinal bacteria

1. **The good ones:** Bifidobacterium bifidum, lactobacillus acidophilus, enterococcus faecalis, bacillus subtilis var. Natto, yeast, and aspergillus. Accounting for 20% of intestinal bacteria, the good bacteria are helpful to stimulate bowel peristalsis, maintain bowel condition, and increase the immunity.

2. **The bad ones:** Staphylococcus, clostridium perfringens, and coliform (toxic strains). Accounting for 10% of intestinal bacteria, these bacteria produce harmful substances including ammonia, hydrogen sulfide, and indole. Dominance by the bad bacteria produces foul-smelling feces and results in reduced immune response and metabolism.

3. **The neutral ones:** Coliform (nontoxic strains) and streptococcus. Accounting for 70% of intestinal bacteria, the neutral bacteria have no specific effect on the body but would join the dominant party of

either the good or the bad bacteria.

A balanced intestinal flora is constituted by 20% of the good bacteria, 10% of the bad bacteria, and 70% of the neutral bacteria. This ratio ensures normal bowel movement and maintains high levels of the immunity. Nevertheless, the increase of the bad bacteria joined by the neutral bacteria causes immediate disturbance to bowel condition, leads to immunodeficiency, and supports cancer development. On the other hand, an excessive amount of the good bacteria may also trigger illnesses, such as Crohn's disease, ulcerative colitis, and hay fever, due to overactivation of the immune system. Hence, it is best to live a balanced lifestyle and keep the balanced proportion of each type of intestinal bacteria.

The consumption of vegetables and fermented foods is very important to a balanced gut environment. Especially in Japan, a country famous for its variety of fermented foods, it is much easier to include these healthy ingredients in our daily meals. There are three reasons why fermented foods are good to our health. **Firstly, fermented foods are rich in the good bacteria, mainly lactobacillus.** Since the good bacteria are helpful to activate the immune system to prevent pathogen invasion, intake of fermented foods is potentially beneficial to the maintenance of bowel condition, immunity improvement, and disease prevention. **Secondly, fermented foods help to activate immune cells in the gut.** Approximately 60% of immune cells are gathered in the intestines, which upon activation contribute greatly to the defense against foreign invasion. **Thirdly, fermented foods are somewhat digested because of microbial activity.** As a result, the digestion of fermented foods requires minimum energy and digestive enzymes, which helps to save the internal resources and build a healthy body.

From ancient times, an abundance of fermented foods like miso, soy sauce, mirin, vinegar, sweet wine, natto, and rice bran pickles has been around in Japanese households. Except for these, western preserved vegetables, kimchi, sauerkraut, cheese, yogurt, wine vinegar, etc. are great sources of fermented foods. For the purpose of intestinal health maintenance and immune enhancement, please be reminded to include some of these foods in your diet.

When Your Immunity Remains Low After Trying Everything

It is an undisputed fact that the immune function

affects our health significantly, which is why we should pay attention to what we eat, make exercise a habit, and try to reduce stress levels. Nevertheless, as our physical and mental functions decrease with age, the immunity exhibits an inevitable decline. Humans are progressing towards death from the moment we were born. Whilst this natural principle can never be violated, to some extent we may control the cause of our demise that awaits us at the end of the day.

As age increases, PD-1 expression on T cells is increased (see Chapter 4, p.107), which leads to T cell deficiency and an unavoidable decline in the immune function. Reduced defense against bacterial or viral invasion potentially raises the risk of geriatric pneumonia. Typically, immune enhancement may be achieved by lifestyle correction, regular exercise, or balanced diet. For elderly people whose immune system could not be boosted effectively, however, hydrogen inhalation offers extra help.

The average life expectancy and the healthy lifespan of the Japanese

1. Male: Average life expectancy: 79.55 years old
   Healthy lifespan: 70.42 years old

Difference: 9.13 years

2. Female: Average life expectancy: 86.30 years old

Healthy lifespan: 73.62 years old

Difference: 12.68 years

(Source: Research performed by the Ministry of Health, Labor and Welfare of Japan in 2010)

Did you know that there is a rough discrepancy of 10 years between the average life expectancy and the healthy lifespan of the Japanese? This 10-year window is defined as *the ailing phase with restricted daily activities.* Many people living through this window are bedridden or dependent on the help of a caregiver. Isn't that a condition quite opposite to a happy ending at the very end of life? The natural process of death involves a decline in mitochondrial function in the previous week and finally leads to the departure in sleep. Hydrogen inhalation helps to maintain high levels of the immunity at an advanced age, and keeps one healthy until reaching the average life expectancy. In that case, hydrogen application could also assist in cutting down a significant portion of medical expenses.

Chapter 6

Return to Work Despite "Having Only Two Months to Live"

Sheltering Cancer Patients, Witnessing Their Recoveries

Hydrogen is a natural substance on Earth, however, this is the first attempt not only in Japan but also in the whole world to apply hydrogen in cancer treatment. In my hospital, stage 4 patients are required to return for regular visits, except for patients admitted for pleural effusion or ascites. Even if diagnosed with metastases, most of my patients are eager to attend periodic appointments, trying to live a normal life. I feel sorry and wish to save those who have continued to seek the cure relentlessly despite being given up by medical institutions. What I want to do is to prolong their lives, and this is the motive for my daily practice.

Nicknamed *the shelter for cancer patients*, my hospital has been providing hydrogen immunotherapy for approximately 400 patients so far. The cases introduced in this chapter are part of the patients who have experienced a remarkable recovery from stage 4 cancer, advanced cancer, or recurrent cancer. Some of them have returned to work in good condition, even though they were once told to "have only two months left." Having said that, it remains difficult to create a positive mindset once you think about the risk of relapse. It is known that few patients achieve a complete recovery even if the tumor has shrunk transiently. By all means would cancer evade the immune system to restart its growth and reproduction.

Only after attempting to apply a variety of antineoplastic drugs did I start to provide hydrogen immunotherapy for patients advised to receive palliative care. It turned out that this treatment approach was successful in lengthening the remaining lifespan from a few months to a couple of years. Nonetheless, for patients experiencing a relapse after life extension, the challenge has just begun. Through patients showing evidence of recurrence, we have discovered a close association between the increase of specialized immune suppressive cells and cancer recurrence. We have also figured out the method to constrain the production of the specific cells. In the near future if everything goes well, curing end-stage cancer patients would no longer be a dream. This has raised a question deep down in my mind as to whether the establishment of hydrogen immunotherapy offers us **a new weapon to conquer diseases and aging**. Lastly, before we go through some of the cases documented until July 2019, please be reminded of the following caveats in order to establish a proper point of view on the efficacy of hydrogen immunotherapy.

The Reading of Tumor Markers

The variation of tumor markers can be displayed in charts based on monthly measurements. Depending on the type of tumor markers, the value is different and varies between individuals, ranging from a number of hundreds to tens of thousands. Overall, the higher the value, the worse the condition.

Similar to share prices, the value of tumor markers fluctuates. After receiving hydrogen immunotherapy, many patients have shown a steady decrease in tumor marker values with slight fluctuations. In the event of a dramatic increase in a tumor marker value, consideration should be given to the possibility of tumor enlargement, or a momentary rise resulted from cancer destruction. With regard to the cases introduced below, fluctuations of tumor marker values were caused by the latter.

Cancer Evaluation Criteria

RECIST and the *WHO* (World Health Organization) guideline are the judging standards commonly used for the evaluation of tumor size and the relative change. According to both criteria, effectiveness is defined as a reduction in tumor size of at least 30%. While RECIST measures the longest dimension, the WHO guideline compares the product (i.e. the area) of the long and short dimensions. As a result, the percentage of tumor reduction acquired by the two criteria differs, and the outcome measured by the WHO standard is supposedly more accurate.

Cancer Remission

Cancer remission is referred to as a temporary or continuous recovery, or alternatively a seemingly vanished condition. Cancer remission can be divided into partial and complete remission. Complete remission (CR) indicates tumor disappearance which lasts longer than one month, whereas partial remission (PR) indicates a 30% or more reduction in tumor volume lasting for more than a month.

In terms of hydrogen immunotherapy, many patients have experienced PR while some are observed close to CR. However, since the risk of recurrence remains high for stage 4 patients even when cancer cells have seemingly disappeared, the treatment shall be continued for patients demonstrating evidence of PR or CR for an extended period.

Therapeutic Hydrogen Inhaler

A variety of hydrogen inhalers have been available in the market nowadays. The picture below shows the machine currently used for hydrogen immunotherapy in my hospital. Patients are allowed to borrow the equipment for home use.

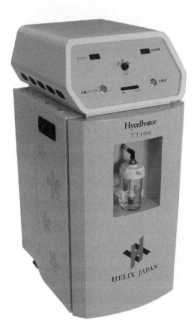

Product Name: Hycellvator ET100
Oxy-hydrogen Output Rate: 1200 ml/min

Clinical Cases of Hydrogen Therapy

Case 1

· Ovarian Cancer (Stage 4) Ms. K·H 33 years old

· Treatment Period: From May 2018 to June 2019

· Surviving at least 13 months

· Treatment Protocol: Hyperthermia Therapy + Low-Dose Antineoplastic Drugs + Hydrogen + Opdivo®

Ms. K·H came to our hospital through the referral of an acquaintance. Now she travels quite a long distance for regular follow-up. When she first arrived, her ovarian tumor had reached a size of more than 10 cm. The tumor was identifiable by palpation and was half filled with liquid. At that time, Ms. K·H could barely stand or walk. After about six months, however, the tumor volume had reduced significantly from 112.93 x 107.07 mm2 to 37.66 x 39.27 mm^2. The reduction rate was calculated as 65.2% according to RECIST criteria (see page 2).

Ms. K·H was initially admitted to our hospital because of the long travel distance. During her stay, she was required to receive hydrogen inhalation for at least 3 hours per day. In May 2018, the value of the tumor marker CA-

125 had decreased from 1600 to 600 in a single month and continued lowering to a level of 252. Yet ongoing treatment was required, given that the normal value should not exceed 35.0. As I have explained repeatedly, continuous recovery is rarely seen despite the fact that tumor reduction and decreased tumor marker values have been observed in 90% of my patients. The percentage of patients managing to maintain sustainable reductions drops to approximately 50%, and thus the treatment must be continued.

From her fresh appearance, Ms. K·H does not give the impression of having cancer. Working on a full recovery, she still travels a long way to our hospital for regular follow-up. Her present treatment protocol involves one-week admission and two-week home care. Besides, Ms. K·H has bought a hydrogen inhaler for home use of over three hours a day.

Case 2

· Lung Cancer (Stage 4)· Ms. H·S 62 years old
· Treatment Period: From June 2014 to June 2019
· Surviving at least 5 years
· Treatment Protocol: Hyperthermia Therapy + Low-Dose Antineoplastic Drugs + Hydrogen + Opdivo®

When she first arrived at our hospital, Ms. H·S was presented with carcinomatous pleuritis, a type of cancer that grows outside the lungs and spreads to the pleura. She was admitted due to an excessive amount of pleural fluid. After the removal of roughly 2 liters of hemorrhagic pleural fluid, her condition remained critical. In situations where carcinomatous pleuritis has arisen from lung cancer, a remaining lifespan of three to fourth months is expected and might be extended up to the maximum of 1 year with the help of medication.

The initial treatment of hyperthermia therapy and low-dose antineoplastic drugs (a smaller amount used to maintain the immunity and stabilize cancer cells) resulted in repetitions of tumor reduction and enlargement (shown in red on the upper left image on page 3). Consequently, Opdivo® and hydrogen were added since February 2016. Ms. H·S also rented a hydrogen inhaler for home use to receive hydrogen inhalation for more than 3 hours per day. From then on, her tumor reduced dramatically, which had almost disappeared in the lower right image on Page 3. Afterwards, Ms. H·S continued to come for outpatient hydrogen immunotherapy and maintained a vigorous and healthy condition. With the application of **hydrogen immunotherapy**, Ms. H·S, who had possibly only three to fourth months left to live, had managed to prolong her life for an additional 5 years and has remained alive until now.

When considering the application of antineoplastic drugs and radiotherapy in the standard of care, *the treatment is deemed effective* for tumor reduction that lasts longer than one month. However, in my opinion, a treatment is only effective when coexistence with cancer or tumor disappearance has continued for more than six months. In this aspect, this is an outstanding case to demonstrate the possibility of 5-year life prolongation for a stage 4 cancer patient. At present, Ms. H·S is close to CR and receives the treatment of Opdivo® once in a month. Even when the tumor vanishes, treatment continuation with extended intervals is still a better approach to cancer recovery. Ms. H·S is a typical example of how tenacious and tough cancer is.

Case 3

· Breast Cancer (Stage 4) / Ms. K·M 46 years old
· Treatment Period: From August 2017 to June 2019
· Surviving at least 22 months
· Treatment Protocol: Hyperthermia Therapy + Low-Dose Antineoplastic Drugs + Hydrogen + Opdivo®

Ms. K·M had axillary and subclavian lymph node metastases when she first visited our hospital. Because surgery was not a feasible therapeutic option for her condition, we had started to add Opdivo® and hydrogen in her treatment course after the application of hyperthermia therapy and low-dose antineoplastic drugs produced little treatment response. Meanwhile, Ms. K·M rented a hydrogen inhaler for home use to receive hydrogen inhalation for over 3 hours per day.

The upper two images shown on page 4 were taken in July 2017. The image in the upper left corner captured the axillary lymph node metastases, while the image in the upper right corner recorded the subclavian lymph node metastases. The scan was performed in a caudal-cephalic direction, which means that the left side of the image represents the right side of the patient, and vice versa. Thus, the metastases were found in the left axillary and subclavian regions.

By contrast, the images taken in April 2018 demonstrated clearly that the left axillary lymph node metastases had almost disappeared, and the subclavian metastases had reduced significantly. At this point, surgery was performed to remove the primary left breast lesion. Since the primary lesion might communicate with the metastatic lesion via cytokines to gain control over the metastases, the removal of the primary lesion helps to decrease the metastatic lesion and leads to better treatment outcome.

Case 4

- Colon Cancer (Recurrence) / Ms. T·K 77 years old
- Treatment Period: From March 2017 to June 2019
- Surviving at least 27 months
- Treatment Protocol: Hyperthermia Therapy + Low-Dose Antineoplastic Drugs + Hydrogen + Opdivo®

Ms. T·K had experienced a local recurrence after surgery, which resulted in the enlargement of the remnant tumor and mediastinal lymph node metastases. Needless to say, most hospitals would choose to apply antineoplastic drugs or radiation therapy for her condition. Nevertheless, she was told that "there is nothing we could do for you."

In the upper left corner on page 5 demonstrated the mediastinal lymph node metastases. The image shown in the upper right corner recorded a massive intrapelvic tumor found at the previous surgical site, which was supposedly the local recurrence developed postoperatively, i.e. infiltration of the intrauterine relapse. Additionally, the value of the tumor marker CA 19-9 had continued to increase.

In March 2017, the tumor marker value was pretty high at around 80 when the application of hyperthermia therapy and low-dose antineoplastic drugs failed to prove its efficacy. Upon our recommendation, Ms. T·K agreed to receive Opdivo® in addition to two-hour outpatient hydrogen inhalation almost daily since May 2018. Because of the treatment, her tumor size had decreased dramatically, so had her tumor marker value reaching less than 35.

Following the treatment of Opdivo® and hydrogen therapy, a swift drop in the tumor marker value indicated tumor reduction in spite of fluctuations. In Ms. T·K's case, the value of CA 19-9 was as high as 235.6 on May 11, a date prior to receiving Opdivo® and hydrogen therapy. The value was 226.5 on June 1, yet a rapid decrease down to 48.7 was documented on July 13. Now the value remains at 22.4, which is within the normal range of below 37.0. Currently, Ms. T·K returns for treatment once a week and continues working as a high school teacher in good health.

Case 5

· Ureteral Cancer (Stage 4) / Mr. K·K 69 years old

· Treatment Period: From October 2016 to June 2019

· Surviving at least 2 years and 8 months

· Treatment Protocol: Hyperthermia Therapy + Low-Dose Antineoplastic Drugs + Hydrogen + Opdivo®

Mr. K·K had ureteral cancer and a metastatic tumor found in his lung. Just like the others, Mr. K·K received outpatient therapy initially and has continued until now. With ongoing treatment, the tumor size is expected to continue shrinking.

In twelve months after the application of hydrogen therapy, the tumor size had reduced from 81.94 x 50.18 mm2 to 41.90 x 53.76 mm^2 (see page 6). Mr. K·K had rented a hydrogen inhaler for home use of more than 3 hours per day. At present, he has continued to receive treatment of Keytruda®—an immune checkpoint inhibitor that has similar effects as Opdivo® and is applicable to NHI for patients with ureteral cancer.

The tumor reduction rate was 34.4% and 45.2% according to RECIST and WHO criteria, respectively. That is, the treatment was considered effective by both criteria since the percentage of tumor reduction was greater than 30%. Although many patients have experienced tumor regrowth subsequent to a decrease in tumor marker value and tumor reduction, an enduring effect is the evidence of proper induction of immune surveillance. Considering that Mr. K·K has experienced stable efficacy, a further reduction of the tumor size is expected with continuous treatment.

Case 6

· Breast Cancer (Recurrence) / Ms. T·M 53 years old
· Treatment Period: From July 2015 to June 2019
· Surviving at least 3 years and 11 months
· Treatment Protocol: Hyperthermia Therapy + Low-Dose Antineoplastic Drugs + Hydrogen

Ms. T·M came to our hospital after having a relapse subsequent to surgery performed by another institution. She was presented with a hard mass in the supraclavicular region covered by reddish and tender skin. The image shown in the upper left corner on page 7 demonstrated the mediastinal lymph node metastases located at the center, while the image shown in the upper right corner indicated the subclavian lymph node metastases.

Due to financial issues, Ms. T·M decided to receive the combined treatment of hyperthermia therapy, low-dose antineoplastic drugs, and hydrogen without Opdivo®. She also rented a hydrogen inhaler for home use of more than 3 hours per day. Opdivo® is considered self-paid medication for all kinds of diseases with the exception of melanoma, non-small cell lung cancer, malignant pleural mesothelioma, renal cell carcinoma, Hodgkin lymphoma, head and neck cancer, and stomach cancer. Since the treatment might cost a fortune, we respect patient autonomy in decision-making contexts as to whether to receive Opdivo® or not.

Regardless of lacking Opdivo®, the images obtained after 30-month treatment demonstrated a gradual reduction of the tumor size. Compared to other cases that had incorporated the treatment of Opdivo®, it was noted that the combination of hydrogen therapy could lead to earlier effects. While Ms. T·M was close to CR, a question was raised as to how much longer should the treatment be continued? The answer is unclear so far, yet it has been suggested that the duration of hydrogen immunotherapy should be extended for at least 3 to 6 months with longer intervals to achieve long-lasting treatment outcome. Similar to annual influenza vaccination, cancer is a much stronger and more unpredictable enemy that necessitates the continuation of immune enhancement. As a result, our protocol is to provide continuous treatment for patients in the future.

Case 7

· Prostate Cancer (Recurrence)/ Mr. S·T 79 years old

· Treatment Period: From March 2018 to June 2019

· Surviving at least 15 months (treatment duration in our hospital)

· Treatment Protocol: Hyperthermia Therapy + Hydrogen

Mr. S·T was diagnosed with prostate cancer. Based on his request, the combination of hyperthermia therapy and hydrogen was provided continuously, at which point he received hydrogen inhalation for 3 to 5 hours per day. Yet, his PSA level had ranged between 30 to 40 without further decrease.

In December 2018, Mr. S·T decided to purchase a hydrogen generator and lengthen the duration of hydrogen inhalation to more than 10 hours a day. "I have decided to bet my life on hydrogen," said Mr. S·T, who had collected much information on hydrogen 1 am determined to "inhale hydrogen for ten hours per day." That was something even

I did not ever consider a reasonable demand, but perhaps a stressful treatment approach. However, it may actually be a possible option if we devide the course into six hours in sleep and two hours each in the morning and the afternoon.

It turned out that his PSA level had decreased from 41.51 to 8.08 within three months, and the current level stayed almost normalized at 5.74. Moreover, the application of surgery or radiotherapy for prostate cancer could lead to problems like erectile dysfunction and

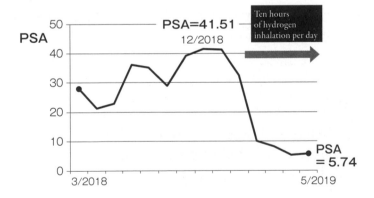

Normalization of the tumor marker level by receiving hydrogen inhalation for ten hours per day

The PSA level was normalized within 5 months after receiving ten hours of hydrogen inhalation per day. The number had decreased from a range between 30 and 40 to 5.74, where the normal value should be less than 5.0.

residual urine. These may be avoided with simplified hydrogen immunotherapy of Opdivo® and hydrogen, which is certainly beneficial to many patients.

Mr. S·T's treatment outcome not only surprised me but also manifested the potential of hydrogen therapy. Currently, we have started to offer a rental service of hydrogen inhalers for prostate cancer patients who are skeptical about Western medicine and prefer to receive hyperthermia therapy only. By providing ten hours of hydrogen therapy per day, we are looking forward to seeing similarly remarkable results. Furthermore, we wish to expand the possibility of curing early-stage prostate cancer with noninvasive treatment measures, such as hydrogen and hyperthermia therapy, other than traditional radiotherapy and antineoplastic drugs.

Case 8

· Pancreatic Cancer (Stage 4) / Ms. M·M 81 years old
· Treatment Period: From October 2018 to June 2019
· Surviving at least 8 months (treatment duration in our hospital)
· Treatment Protocol: Hyperthermia Therapy + Low-Dose Antineoplastic Drugs + Hydrogen + Opdivo®

We had provided hydrogen immunotherapy for Ms. M·M in order to treat her advanced pancreatic cancer, and it turned out that the tumor volume had reduced 52.4% in three months, as shown on page 8. Ms. M·M also purchased a hydrogen inhaler to receive at least 3 hours of hydrogen inhalation daily at home. Given her advanced age and a relatively short treatment course of 8 months, close monitoring was necessary. However, it is noteworthy that even for pancreatic cancer, which is usually associated with poor prognosis, the tumor size had been reduced dramatically without side effects. Hydrogen immunotherapy had been effective in maintaining the quality of life and extending the remaining lifespan for Ms. M·M.

Even though Ms. M·M was admitted due to loss of appetite every now and then, she always managed to recover after one week's stay. Just like her case, I have a strong feeling that hydrogen immunotherapy would help to prolong the lives of patients diagnosed with stage 4 pancreatic cancer for a couple of years without producing any significant side effects.

Chapter 7

Hydrogen Prolongs Healthy Lifespan by 10 Years

Reaching the Average Life Expectancy in Good Health

While the average life expectancy is referred to as the length of our lives, the healthy lifespan indicates the time span for us to have a normal life without physical restraints. The difference between the average life expectancy and the healthy lifespan is approximately 10 years, during which almost every living person becomes bedridden or requires to be taken care of by a caregiver. The main causes of this disparity may include geriatric pneumonia, dementia, brain infarction, and cancer, which are somehow connected to immune abnormalities. Since disease development is highly associated with the immune response, **boosting the immunity from our daily lives is helpful to reach the average life expectancy in good health.**

Loss of appetite and reduced motor function are commonly seen in elderly people who are diagnosed with these disorders. Physical inactivity and a persistent indoor lifestyle potentially lead to disuse syndrome[†] and muscle atrophy, which eventually results in a bedridden condition for many patients. Besides, it should be noted that a bone fracture is a typical cause for bedridden older people. But most importantly, the above-mentioned diseases should be prevented to further avoid a bedridden condition.

Supposedly, hydrogen inhalation helps to achieve immune enhancement and consequently prolongs the average life expectancy by more than 10 years. This raises the number of people reaching the age of 100 and more, while the increase of healthy senior citizens lowers the burden of national healthcare expenses. In addition, hydrogen is beneficial to improve the quality of life for the elderly population.

† Disuse syndrome is a condition in which a person experiences a decline in motor function which limits physical activity and leads to other causes of discomfort.

Hydrogen Application Prevents Dementia

Dementia is a disease caused by brain dysfunction. According to the Ministry of Health, Labor and Welfare of Japan, the number of people living with dementia is estimated to reach 7.3 million in Japan by 2025. This is equal to an incidence of one in five elderly residents. Thus, it is highly likely that our own loved ones would suffer from dementia.

There are several types of dementia, mainly including Alzheimer's disease, dementia with Lewy bodies, and vascular dementia. Alzheimer's disease and dementia with Lewy bodies are characterized by the deposition of an abnormal protein within the brain that damages the neuron, whereas vascular dementia is caused by brain cell impairment resulted from cerebrovascular obstruction and breakage. Cellular damage in the brain is the primary cause of brain dysfunction, memory loss, and emotional instability that are observed in these types of dementia. Additional symptoms may include wandering, hallucination, and hostility, which impose not just physical and financial burdens but also an emotionally overwhelming task on the family.

To date, there has been no effective and comprehensive treatment for dementia. However, we have discovered information about the prevention and improvement of mild cognitive impairment (MCI—a pre-dementia state with ongoing alteration of the brain function) in an experiment. Twenty subjects including males and females aged between 60 to 70 had participated in this study. The subjects had shown normal cognitive function in dementia tests, and were asked to inhale hydrogen five times per day. After two weeks, it was suggested that the cerebral control function was improved. Meanwhile, the levels of three types of protein associated with MCI risks varied in hematology test, demonstrating an anti-inflammatory effect to the brain. Hence, **we believe that hydrogen application is effective in reducing the risk of MCI as well as alleviating the symptoms of dementia.**

Alzheimer's Disease Can Be Prevented via the Prevention of Intracerebral Oxidation

It has been proven that Alzheimer's disease reduces the number of cerebral neurons, leading to an overall atrophy of cerebral tissues focusing on *hippocampus* that is in charge of the memory function. *Neurofibrillary tangles* that appear as thread-like structures have been shown in cerebral neurons found in patients with Alzheimer's disease. Alzheimer's disease is characterized by the deposition of β-amyloid protein in the brain, which induces neuronal alteration and dislodgment, decreases cerebral function, and develops cerebral atrophy.

However, a recent study revealed that the actual cause of Alzheimer's disease is the linkage between β-amyloid protein and intracerebral receptors. Following the combination of β-amyloid protein and intracerebral receptors, lipids—the major component of the brain tissue—start to degrade as the level of ROS increases. This reaction results in neuronal destruction and gives rise to Alzheimer's disease. In other words, Alzheimer's disease is mainly caused by intracerebral oxidation.

It has been reported in animal experiments that hydrogen application in mice is effective in inhibiting memory impairment accompanied by memory loss and inflammation. Selective removal of the bad ROS by hydrogen is highly beneficial to the prevention of Alzheimer's disease. Moreover, evidence points out that T cells with PD-1 expression are related to dementia. As we have known, PD-1 molecules are automatically expressed on activated T cells to prevent the immune system from overreacting. By combining with PD-1 molecules, Opdivo® relieves the immunosuppression to assist in cancer treatment.

Nevertheless, according to our observation, Opdivo® is also effective in dementia treatment. In fact, promising scores of the Hasegawa Dementia Scale† that are considered indications of symptom improvement were recorded in older patients who received hydrogen inhalation. Hydrogen is useful in activating fatigued T cells with PD-1 expression, and therefore it may potentially produce a remarkable effect on dementia treatment and prevention in the future.

> † Hasegawa Dementia Scale is a commonly used screening tool for dementia, which was established by the Japanese pioneer, Dr. Kazuo Hasegawa.

Hydrogen Is a Promising Hope for Treatment of Parkinson's Disease

Parkinson's disease is induced by the aggregation of *Lewy bodies*—proteins surrounded by neurofibrillary tangles—in the nerves. The pathogenesis of Parkinson's disease involves neuronal disturbance resulted from the production of ROS by Lewy bodies. Parkinson's disease is typically seen in the age group of 50 to 60 and it affects more men than women. The most common symptoms of Parkinson's disease may include *tremor*, *rigidity* (muscle contraction and stiff joints), *bradykinesia* (slow or reduced movement), and *postural instability* (increased risk of falls).

There is a patient in our hospital who had given up on golf for 8 years because of the tremors caused by Parkinson's disease. After he started to receive hydrogen inhalation for one hour per day, and occasionally one hour each in the morning and the evening, his symptom was improved in one year. Recently, he has resumed the habit of playing golf on weekends and enjoys it very much. He is actually living proof that hydrogen helps to repair damaged brain neurons. Furthermore, inhibition of ROS contributes substantially to the prevention and improvement of Parkinson's disease.

Hydrogen Facilitates Stroke Treatment and Prevention

The breakage of cerebral vessels is called "cerebral hemorrhage," while the blockage of these vessels is referred to as "cerebral infarction." The combination of cerebral hemorrhage and cerebral infarction is known as "stroke." Stroke is the fourth leading cause of death in Japan following cardiac diseases and pneumonia. Additionally, stroke is a primary cause of a large number of bedridden patients.

Stroke is induced by vascular aging. The continual deterioration of arteriosclerosis results in vascular stenosis, which in turn increases blood pressure and the risks of vessel breakage and embolism. Since arteriosclerosis is deeply connected to the bad ROS that is removable by hydrogen, it is possible to prevent vascular aging and consequent onset of stroke through routine hydrogen inhalation. Moreover, hydrogen is a powerful tool in treating cerebral infarction. Once cerebral vessels are obstructed, oxygen transport is impeded to induce neuronal necrosis and inflammation in a short time. When the cerebral blood flow is resumed by treatment, a significant amount of the bad ROS would be generated due to existing inflammatory condition.

A high level of the bad ROS damages and oxidizes the brain cells. Yet, the combination of the bad ROS with nitric oxide generated by macrophages or neutrophils gathering at the inflammatory site produces an even more potent oxidant—peroxynitrite—and leads to severe tissue impairment. Overall, in the event of cerebral infarction, the cerebral cells would be harmed by the effect of the bad ROS produced when the blood flow resumes after treatment as well as by the generation of peroxynitrite at the inflammatory site.

Nevertheless, the bad ROS can be inhibited via hydrogen inhalation to reduce neuronal damage in the brain. It has been identified that when treating patients with acute cerebral infarction, co-administration of hydrogen and edaravone results in better treatment outcome than edaravone monotherapy. With its small molecular size, hydrogen can be delivered into cells independent of the vascular system and is expected to exhibit superior effects compared to a variety of medicines.

The Significance of Hydrogen in Myocardial Infarction Treatment and Prevention

Myocardial infarction is a condition caused by vascular aging of the cardiac muscle. Vascular aging is the precursor of arteriosclerosis, which gives rise to vascular stenosis and stagnant flow. The final outcome is the development of myocardial necrosis and infarction. Similar to stroke, the course of arteriosclerosis in cardiac vessels is closely related to the bad ROS, and therefore can be effectively prevented by hydrogen.

The current treatment options for myocardial

infarction primarily include *coronary artery bypass graft* and *coronary angioplasty*. In contrast to the creation of an alternative vascular route by the former, coronary angioplasty involves the insertion of a balloon or stent (a metallic mesh tube) to achieve lumen dilatation. In recent years, coronary angioplasty has become a more popular choice for cardiac patient, though a restenosis rate of 30% has been reported.

Specifically, intimal inflammation resulted from the insertion of foreign bodies such as a balloon or stent is the leading cause of restenosis, where intimal hyperplasia and thrombosis brings about re-narrowing of the lumen. The expansion of inflammation is strongly associated with the bad ROS, which is generated in the intima as an immune response to foreign body insertion. An excessive amount of the bad ROS induces unnecessary inflammation and leads to restenosis.

However, it has been shown in mice experiments that hydrogen application inhibits restenosis induced by inflammatory response. Through further research, it is perhaps possible to *consider hydrogen as the first-line treatment for myocardial infarction* in the near future.

Hydrogen Soothes Myalgia and Arthralgia

Across generations, many people have been affected by symptoms of myalgia, including neck and shoulder stiffness and low back pain. Arthralgia involving shoulders, knees, or ankles is another common issue for modern people. Hydrogen is useful in analgesic treatment for orthopedic patients. Similar to the anti-inflammatory agents, analgesics, and steroids used in the Department of Pain Management and Department of Orthopedics, hydrogen inhibits inflammation via chemical reactions. However, hydrogen is superior to medications in terms of the suitability for whole-body use, side effects and dosage limits. So, what exactly is the mechanism of pain relief by hydrogen? Firstly, the sensation of pain is generated by the process described below.

Generation of pain

1. Induction of chain reactions in multiple cytokines (a general term for proteins released by cells to interact with specific cells) by certain stimulation
2. Inflammatory substances are released by an enzyme to cause inflammation.
3. Inflammation is detected by sensory nerves, giving

rise to the sensation of pain.

Most of the anti-inflammatory agents, analgesics, and steroids are designed to prevent cyclooxygenase (COX), the enzyme involved in step 2, from communicating cytokine reactions to inflammatory substances. Thus, withdrawal results in worsening of inflammation and pain. By contrast, hydrogen inhibits one of the NF-κB factors—the ROS—in a state earlier than step 2 to achieve an analgesic effect. Besides, hydrogen can be administered via intramuscular or joint injection for pain management. Hydrogen leads to dull pain in areas accumulated by the ROS, which is soon followed by a sense of warmth and a dramatic reduction in pain.

In comparison to medications, hydrogen exerts similar anti-inflammatory effects without causing any side effects. Moreover, hydrogen is suitable for whole-body use without dosage limits. Except for use in myalgia or arthralgia for the general population, hydrogen may be beneficial to muscle and joint care for sportsmen and sportswomen.

Hydrogen Works Through the Same Pathway as Sirtuin Genes (Longevity Genes)

The sirtuin gene (SIRT1) is one of the longevity genes that slow down the aging process. The function of sirtuin genes is to protect the *telomeres* located at the ends of chromosomes and to improve cell health. The *telomeres* are designed to shorten with each round of cell division until they reach a critical length, at which point the cells can no longer undergo any process of division and may become potentially cancerous. Thus, the cells must go through a strictly regulated cell suicide process known as programmed cell death, or apoptosis.

Nevertheless, activation of sirtuin genes helps to protect the telomeres, promote cell health, and delay the aging process. Additional advantages of sirtuin activation include ROS removal, cancer prevention, as well as obesity and diabetes improvement. Moreover, activation of PGC-1α (substance inhibiting gene transcription) by sirtuin genes facilitates mitochondrial production and function. In detail, sirtuin genes achieve mitochondrial activation through the following steps.

1. Activation of sirtuin genes by exercise or fasting

2. Increase of PGC-1α function

3. Increase of mitochondrial production and function

On the other hand, hydrogen activates mitochondria through a similar pathway. As described below, hydrogen boosts mitochondrial function via direct activation of PGC-1α.

1. Activation of PGC-1α by hydrogen

2. Increase of mitochondrial production and function

While PGC-1α activation can be achieved by both sirtuin genes and hydrogen, the simplified process involved in hydrogen application is supposed to enhance mitochondrial function more efficiently. Even though this is what we know for now, further research may help to expand hydrogen application through this pathway.

An Age-Related Decline in Mitochondrial Function Is Observed in Males Since Age 42

Basically, a reduction in mitochondrial function begins to occur in the age of 40 to 50. Many people in this age group start to experience a decline in physical function, reduced energy level, weight gain, and body discomfort. This shift is attributed to many factors and varies between individuals. Nonetheless, it is true that the mechanism of energy production changes with age.

While we are young, the body relies on the *glycolytic system* to produce abundant energy rapidly by consuming glucose. That is why young people always appear energized despite staying up late. For the same reason, youngsters maintain a fixed figure even with occasional indulgence in food and drinks. When we grow older, our bodies depend on the *mitochondrial energy generating system (MEGS)* for energy production via oxygen consumption. Therefore, keeping the same dietary habit and lifestyle as before usually leads to discomfort. Complaints about tiredness, difficulty to lose weight, and "an unfamiliar feeling about one's own body" are often heard among the middle-aged group. A signal perhaps, such a sense may be an implication that the current route of energy production is in conflict with your longstanding style of living.

The glycolytic system is dedicated to producing instant muscular power as required in a sprint race, whereas the MEGS is intended to generate long-lasting energy supportive of a marathon game. Compared to the glycolytic system, the efficiency of the MEGS is 16 times higher, which enables stable energy output. After reaching middle age, it is recommended to perform aerobic exercise, such as walking, swimming, jogging, cycling, and yoga, and to adopt dietary habits and lifestyles detailed in Chapter 5 to activate the MEGS.

In Japan, the year in which alteration in physical functioning occurs is called "yakudoshi" (meaning a calamitous year). Starting from age 42, physiological changes take place with the aging process. During the age of 40 to 50, lifestyle correction involving dietary habits, exercise and daily schedule is beneficial to the activation of the MEGS. This helps to prevent metabolic syndrome encompassing hyperlipidemia, hyperglycemia, and hypertension caused by visceral obesity, and leads to a healthy and independent life to the age of 70 or 80.

Remove Excess Fat and Maintain a Slim Body

Mitochondrial activation is substantially beneficial to our health after we reach the age of 40 to 50. As mentioned above, mitochondrial activation is good for the prevention and improvement of metabolic syndrome. In addition, hydrogen is helpful in the removal of extra fat and the promotion of a healthy, slim body shape. Yet, the key factor of this lies in the reorganization of bowel condition.

In the human gut reside *Firmicutes*, bacteria that favor a predisposition to obesity, and *Bacteroidetes*, bacteria that promote weight loss. Obviously, an increase of the latter helps to prevent obesity in a healthy way. On the one hand, *Firmicutes* facilitate food breakdown, digestion, and energy storage. Because of methane production and inhibition of intestinal peristalsis, *Firmicutes* are linked to smelly flatulence and constipation. On the other hand, *Bacteroidetes* generate short-chain fatty acids, which speed up fat burning and decrease fat storage. As a result, a lower Firmicutes/Bacteroidetes ratio in the bowel is significantly favorable for obesity prevention.

Moreover, Bacteroidetes produce hydrogen within the body. Equal to the substance we inhale in, hydrogen produced inside the body is helpful to prevent hazards derived from the ROS and inhibit oxidative processes. Since Bacteroidetes multiply and prosper through the consumption of dietary fiber, intake of burdock, dried radish, asparagus, and soya bean increases the amount of Bacteroidetes. Besides, Bacteroidetes thrive on a lower Oxidation-Reduction Potential (ORP). The ORP reading is a measurement that indicates the tendency towards oxidation or reduction (the opposite process of oxidation) in a given environment. It has been demonstrated that hydrogen inhalation decreases the ORP reading of the intestinal milieu, and therefore increases the level of Bacteroidetes to assist in weight loss.

Stress Reduction—Reducing the Origin of Diseases

It is now commonly known that stress is harmful to our health. And it is a fact that many cancer patients have experienced tremendously stressful events in the previous years. According to a report from the Centers for Disease Control and Prevention (CDC) of the US, 90% of diseases are connected with stress. Stress is generally considered a psychological burden resulted from interpersonal relationships with colleagues, family, and friends. However, this accounts for merely a part of the stressors. A comprehensive list of our daily stressors is provided as below.

Sources of Stressors

· Physical Stressor: Temperature change, noise, dryness, humidity, etc.
· Social Stressor: Occupational or financial changes, interpersonal relationships, etc.
· Psychological and Emotional Stressor: Nervousness, agitation, worry, anxiety, loneliness, anger, rage, etc.
· Physiological Stressor: Fatigue, insomnia, health impairment, infection, etc.

(Source: an excerpt from the webpage of the Japanese Association of Preventive Medicine for Adult Disease)

Our physical and mental functions vary upon exposure to these stressors, which is the cause of stress. Originally, stress is produced to fight against the stressor for survival out of necessity. Chronic stress, however, gives rise to a series of deleterious effects to the body, leading to problems like migraines, gastritis, gastric ulcers, hypertension, myocardial infarction, stroke, cancer, constipation, diarrhea, allergies, and depression. In this modern era, it is rather difficult to identify an illness that has no association with stress.

To prevent and improve disorders arisen from stress, the best solution is to get rid of the stressor. Nevertheless, exclusion of stressful situations at workplace or home is not an easy task. Although I have been trying to advise patients to cultivate a hobby for daily stress relief, I have also received a reply that "I don't really have hobbies" from many people. Perhaps it is just uneasy to escape from stress for many of us.

Once stress is formed, *anti-stress hormone* is secreted by the adrenal cortex to mitigate the influence, while the bad ROS is produced at the same time. As a result, chronic stress brings about considerable accumulation of the bad ROS, which induces diseases including gastric ulcers, gastritis, myocardial infarction, stroke, and cancer. Hydrogen application interrupts this vicious cycle through the inhibition of the bad ROS and the reduction of cellular oxidation, which assist in the prevention and improvement of various disorders resulted from stress.

Furthermore, with a duration longer than 30 minutes, hydrogen inhalation induces the generation of theta wave to achieve a meditative state, which is most suitable for stress relief. Thus, it is important to receive hydrogen inhalation once per day to acquire mental tranquility. If you don't have the right time or right interest for stress reduction, it might be good for you to relieve your daily stress via hydrogen inhalation.

Chapter 8

The Era of Customized Treatment Approaches

"Optimal Medicine" Is the Evolved Version of Integrative Medicine

Currently, healthcare services provided in medical facilities are primarily *symptomatic treatment* established on the basis of modern Western medicine, which focuses on healing illnesses and relieving symptoms. Recently however, a novel idea centering on *causal treatment* of the physical and mental aspects, which requires the application of traditional or alternative medicine, has been slowly adopted by the medical field to displace the goal of disease treatment. *Integrative medicine* combines the major feature of both symptomatic treatment and causal treatment to offer the most adequate *customized treatment approaches* to every patient. Likewise, *hydrogen immunotherapy* which integrates a complex of diverse immunotherapies is considered an example of customized treatment approaches.

Nevertheless, the shortcoming of integrative medicine lies in a lack of clinically significant evidence or scientific basis. That is, it is unclear how integrative medicine benefits the body even if it is "effective." From an immunological perspective, there are plenty of complementary and alternative therapies in the field of integrative medicine, such as yoga, aromatherapy, acupuncture, homeopathy, mental/psychological treatment, and dietary treatment. Yet supposedly, these methods work by promoting the immunity. Based on this proposition, we have continued to analyze immune parameters collected from research with the aim of establishing supportive evidence for integrative medicine.

The forthcoming focus in the ever-evolving world of medicine is *precision medicine*, interchangeably known as *optimal medicine* or *personalized medicine*. Combining hyperthermia therapy, low-dose antineoplastic drugs, hydrogen, and Opdivo®, *hydrogen immunotherapy* conducted in our hospital is one of the most effective treatment options for patients. In particular, the integration of hyperthermia therapy and low-dose antineoplastic drugs utilizes a relatively high temperature to reduce the dosage to one third or one fourth of the typical dose. This approach is useful in activating the immune system, achieving massive destruction of cancer cells, and inducing the so-called immunogenic cell death.

Through the study of case collections since 2016, we have discovered the fact that hydrogen improves the outcome of immunotherapies significantly. Although we have not started gathering practical proof, we have collected over four hundred cases to demonstrate the efficacy of hydrogen immunotherapy. From now on, I intend to investigate immunological evidence of treatments like yoga, aromatherapy, acupuncture, homeopathy, and mental/psychological treatment, in order to apply these methods accordingly. The inclusion and customization of these therapies based on individual condition lead the quickest way towards precision medicine. This is the medical evolution and the optimal, personalized medicine we shall seek in a real sense.

In 2018, an epochal article published in the international academic journal, *Nature Medicine*, revealed the possibility of saving terminal cancer patients with immunotherapy only. The treatment approach reported in this paper was on immune cell therapy, which aimed to recognize and destroy cancer cells by identifying the cancer antigen/marker presented in breast cancer patients. Additionally, Opdivo® was used to lift the immunosuppression. Cancer antigens are special proteins expressed on cancer cells and they are identified as "foreign substances" by the immune system. Upon identification, cancer antigens trigger the immune system to launch the attack against cancer cells. The treatment approach mentioned above, albeit reported as a type of immunotherapy, involved the induction of the most potent lymphocytes against the specific cancer antigen presented in the patient, as well as the co-administration of Opdivo®. From a patient's point of view, this is the best practice of precision medicine.

Japanese medicine is divergent in every sense. While the long-standing practice of mainstream Western medicine helps to restrain metabolic syndrome including hypertension, diabetes, and hyperlipidemia temporarily, it does not aid in fundamental treatments. Specifically, cancer is the most common disease in Japan. In spite of medical advancement, the number of cancer patients has continued to raise. Although Western medicine has been proven powerless to resolve advanced cancers, it happens that integrative medicine has been in transition. For many years, the main concern about integrative medicine has always been the unsettled scarcity of evidence. To avoid misunderstanding, integrative medicine should be described as a treatment approach that works by activating and adjusting the immunity from time to time, in order to maintain proper immune function for the best treatment outcome.

The Immunity Helps to Raise the Natural Self-Healing Ability of Our Bodies

The immune system has two major functions: recognition and removal of harmful foreign substances. Foreign invaders, such as pathogens or toxic dusts in the air, and bacteria or viruses in the food, exist in our daily lives, not to mention malignant cells formed inside our bodies. Without proper identification and elimination of these foreign materials, our bodies are easily corrupted by bacterial, viral, and cancerous proliferation. Yet, the immune system does not launch any attack immediately upon recognition of foreign bodies. In addition, it would be problematic to misidentify normal structures as targets. A malfunctioning, overactive immune system triggers abnormal immune responses under normal condition, leading to allergic disorders including rheumatism, collagen disease, and hay fever.

Take hay fever for example. Pollen allergens are not harmful to the body, and thus people without hay fever do not experience allergic reactions after inhaling pollen. By contrast, once exposed to pollen by eyes and nose, the immune system of people suffering from hay fever recognizes the "foreign substances" and produces

IgE (Immunoglobulin E) antibodies straight away. IgE antibodies are generated along with each exposure and accumulate on the nasal mucosa. When reaching a certain amount, symptoms like sneezes, runny nose, and stuffy nose would be elicited to expel initially unharmful pollen allergens.

This is my personal opinion. Ranging from AMPK (AMP-activated protein kinase that maintains glucose and lipid homeostasis), sirtuin genes (longevity genes), PGC-1α, to mitochondrial signaling pathways, the energy sensors in our bodies are also responsible for positive and negative regulation of these structures. As a result, overactivation of the immune system is potentially close related to mitochondria, and could be modulated by hydrogen.

Not only is hydrogen helpful to mitigate infections, cancer, and dementia that arise from immune deficiency, it is also beneficial to disorders resulted from immune overreaction, including hay fever, ulcerative colitis, and Crohn's disease. Thus, hydrogen inhalation on a daily basis maintains the normal function of the immune system even at an advanced age and promotes healthy longevity.

Simplify Surgical Procedures by Hydrogen Immunotherapy

In terms of cancer treatment, it has been believed so far that surgical tumor removal is the best solution, and lymph nodes must be resected completely. Regarding unsuccessfully resected advanced cancer, the mainstream approach is suppression by the use of antineoplastic drugs. Yet this trend has been changing somewhat.

In the past, extended surgery aimed for large-scale tumor removal was the primary option. However, similar results were shown in a report comparing gastric cancer patients who had and had not undergone extended surgery. This became an opportunity that shifted the preference of extended surgery towards minimally invasive operations.

Previously, it was thought that the removal of cancerized organs and the surrounding lymph nodes matters the most. Thus, it was said that *the prognosis relies on the performance of large-scale lymph node resection*. Especially for gastric cancer, the golden rule was *the wider the lymph node resection, the better the prognosis*. However, there has been no randomized controlled trial (RCT)—the most reliable research method—conducted in relation to this concept in Japan. The only RCT, implemented in the Netherlands, did not acknowledge a significant association between lymph node clearance (surgical removal of lymph node metastases) and prognosis. Although a few issues had been noted in this RCT concerning the disparity in surgical techniques and physiques between Japanese and Dutch people, it seems unnecessary to completely remove the lymph nodes in consideration of the RCT result showing no significant difference from extended clearance for gastric cancer. Instead, the performance of partial resection that leaves residual tissues to induce the immunity might lead to a higher success rate.

In particular, doctors have begun preserving lymph nodes to achieve higher immune activity post-surgically. Lymph nodes are designed to screen for traces of bacteria, virus, or cancer cells existing in the lymph passing through the lymph vessels. They are the structures that trigger immune activation. In other words, lymph nodes are tiny organs filled with cancer cells and immune cells where the immune system is most active. Hence, hydrogen inhalation before and after surgery could achieve immune activation through remnant lymph nodes to help with relapse prevention and life prolongation.

Furthermore, surgery is a procedure involving partial organ removal, and therefore functional impairment is expected to occur correspondingly. For instance, patients receiving gastrectomy have commonly exhibited reduced food intake. Symptoms of palpitations, dizziness, and fatigue brought on by dumping syndrome (general symptoms arisen from food moving too quickly from the stomach to the duodenum) are also distressing for many people. While the impact is dependent on the surgical extent, the performance of lung resection inevitably leads to a decline in lung function and even reduced motor function. In the case of colon resection, larger surgical extent can cause frequent bowel movements or diarrheal stool, whereas an artificial anus is required when the lesion of rectal cancer is close to the anus. In conclusion, the postoperative quality of life is typically suboptimal for patients undergone organ resection.

But then, surgery is an element of the standard of care for cancer treatment, an traditional yet reliable way to remove cancer tissues directly. Apart from long-standing open surgery, endoscopic surgery has gained popularity due to reduced physical burden to the patient. During different operative procedures, the patient's blood flow may be ceased temporarily, During different operative procedures, the patient's blood flow may be ceased temporarily. And when the blood flow is resumed, a significant amount of ROS is produced. With regard to open surgery, it is proposed that upon exposure to oxygen in the air, ROS is generated so as dramatic oxidative stress by organs used to functioning in low levels of oxygen.

ROS can be divided into two groups: the good ROS and the bad ROS. Though the good ROS causes no harm to the body, the co-produced bad ROS promotes oxidative processes and lowers the immunity. A major characteristic of hydrogen is to keep the good ROS and eliminate only the bad ROS. In addition, hydrogen activates fatigued mitochondria that are formed because of pain or hospitalization to reinvigorate T cells for immune enhancement.

In the coming years, hydrogen may be applied before and after operative procedures which emphasize the removal of primary lesions and the preservation of lymph nodes. Such an approach not only simplifies surgical procedures, but also reduces surgical duration, and hence decreases complications and length of stay. Most importantly, it improves the postoperative quality of life as well as the postoperative survival for the patients.

Hydrogen Reduces Damage Caused by Radiotherapy and Antineoplastic Drugs

As part of the standard of care, radiotherapy is a procedure that uses radiation such as X-ray, γ-ray, and cathode ray to inhibit cancer proliferation or to kill cancer cells. One of the major advantages of radiotherapy is reduced physical burdens compared to surgical procedures that require tissue removal. Yet, the disadvantages of radiotherapy may include lower efficacy and multiple side effects, including fatigue, loss of appetite, nausea, diarrhea, and hair loss. These are caused by a direct interaction of radiation with the body, or an indirect interaction between ROS produced by the incident radiation and normal cells. However, hydrogen inhalation before and after radiotherapy facilitates the clearance of the bad ROS, which is effective in reducing the side effects.

Likewise, hydrogen lessens the intensity of side effects arising from antineoplastic treatment, another component of the standard of care, which hinders cancer proliferation or destroys cancer cells by medication. In recent years, the development of potent agents has been very helpful to cancer treatment, especially for early cancer. Nonetheless, antineoplastic drugs also affect normal cells and produce ROS. During antineoplastic treatment, many patients have suffered from side effects such as general fatigue, loss of appetite, and intense nausea, which can be significantly alleviated by hydrogen inhalation.

Moreover, hydrogen exerts similar effects against cisplatin-induced renal toxicity. Cisplatin is a versatile antineoplastic agent that can be used in lung, stomach, esophageal, bladder, prostate, ovarian, and cervical cancers, as well as malignant lymphoma. However, cisplatin treatment brings about serious side effects, particularly nephrotoxicity. As a result, the drawback of cisplatin is dosage limits which vary between individuals. Unsurprisingly, ROS is the culprit for cisplatin-induced renal injury. Once renal mitochondria are damaged by cisplatin, a great number of ROS is generated to oxidize renal cells. Additionally, antioxidant production within the body is decreased by cisplatin in order to remove ROS and hence significant renal damage is caused.

Another good example of reduced side effects through hydrogen inhalation is oxaliplatin—an antineoplastic agent for gastric and colorectal cancer. Commonly reported side effects of oxaliplatin include peripheral neuropathy like numbness in the feet or hands, and severe peripheral neuropathy which affects the ability of walking, writing, self-feeding, and lowers the quality of life significantly. The occurrence of side effects leads to treatment suspension, whereas treatment resumption after certain time diminishes the treatment effect. And again, ROS generated by drug administration is one of the main causes of these side effects. Massive ROS production forces mitochondria to release cytochrome c to induce apoptosis. Peripheral neuropathy occurs when neurons in the spinal cord react to cytochrome c and undergo cellular suicide. However, it is possible to prevent neuronal suicide and to mitigate side effects of oxaliplatin by removing the bad ROS with hydrogen inhalation. In addition, a reduction in side effects is favorable for continuous drug administration and better treatment outcome.

In comparison to the standard of care, hydrogen therapy is a gentler treatment approach to offer similar outcomes with lesser side effects. In the coming years, if patients are allowed to choose the treatment method suitable for their physical condition, not only may the quality of life be maintained, but the life expectancy may also be extended. I am looking forward to this upcoming era of customized treatment approaches, for which the preparation and deployment have been started in my hospital.

Achieve Healthy Longevity via Mitochondria

Mitochondria, the energy factory of the body, can be activated by hydrogen to further energize T cells to launch immediate attack upon identifying foreign invaders, keeping the normal function of the immune system. Mitochondria are organelles found in most cells that are responsible for energy production needed for our own survival. That is to say, our lives are dependent on adequate energy supply by healthy mitochondria. On the other hand, mitochondrial dysfunction results in energy reduction and immune deficiency.

Have you ever wondered how well your mitochondrial function is? If this is measurable, to some extent it is possible to predict personal predispositions to various diseases like cancer and infection. While the examination of mitochondrial function has not been established, it is suggested that mitochondria might aid in disease or prognosis prediction in the near future. Similarly, there has been a lack of effectiveness indicators for prophylactic treatment. Through the examination of mitochondrial function, however, it is possible to gain a clearer understanding of treatment potency. Apart from cancer treatment, assessment of mitochondrial function is an epoch-making achievement to the entire medical world.

Mitochondria can almost be found in each of the 4 trillion cells constituting the human body, to produce sufficient energy for our survival. While energy supply is dominated by the glycolytic system in younger people, the mitochondrial energy generating system (MEGS) takes charge of energy production after the age of 40 to 50. With an efficiency 16 times higher than the glycolytic system, stable energy output of the MEGS inhibits ROS to prevent the body from "rusting." In order to achieve mitochondrial activation and take advantage of the MEGS, it is important to perform aerobic exercise, consume ingredients rich in CoQ10, and try to lower your stress levels.

Vigorous mitochondria help to activate immune cells, promote the attack against foreign substances, and protect our health. As we have mentioned earlier, hydrogen is one of the powerful elements for mitochondrial activation. In addition to cancer immunotherapy, hydrogen is beneficial to health improvement, longevity, anti-aging, and weight loss. It is my hope to bring more people to experience the advantage brought on by hydrogen and to further improve the quality of life for everyone.

Conclusion

Almost every patient in our hospital suffers from end-stage cancer. Before they came to us, most of them had failed to respond to various treatments and were given up on by other medical institutions. The following is an intriguing excerpt from a survey conducted by a newspaper called "Chunichi Shimbun" that revealed a significant divergence in the perspective of doctors and patients in terms of cancer treatment.

- · Question: Are you willing to fight against cancer till the end?
- · Answer: 90% of the patients and 18% of the doctors participated in this survey reported that they are willing to do so.
- · Question: How would you like to face your demise?
- · Answer: 95% of the patients and 51% of the doctors reported that they wish to pass on after trying all available treatments.

That is the real difference between the two parties. Patients desire to receive treatment no matter what it takes, whereas doctors do not hold such a strong belief, and tend to give up on patients at the end. This results in a number of six hundred thousand cancer refugees who are seeking the appropriate treatment and trying to find a slim chance of survival on their own. In our hospital, we have provided hydrogen immunotherapy for them, and we have successfully prolonged their remaining life expectancy— *as short as two months*—for another 1 to 3 years. We have been working with patients and managed to increase their immunity to achieve life prolongation.

Lastly, please do not lose hope. The standard of care— surgery, antineoplastic drugs, and radiotherapy—is not the only approach to cancer treatment. In fact, there are many other ways to combat cancer, by which many people have been able to survive longer. It is my intention to provide correct information about effective treatments for patients living with terminal cancer. I do hope that this book would serve as a source of hope for many cancer refugees to help them find the way to live longer.

Written in July 2019 by Junji Akagi
Superintendent of Tamana Regional Health Medical
Center, Kumamoto Kenhoku Hospital

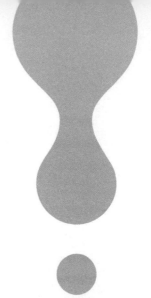

臺灣氫分子
醫療促進協會

Taiwan Association for the Promotion of Molecular Hydrogen.

→ Our Missions

1. To Create a Platform for Industry, Academia, and Government Collaboration on Hydrogen Medicine
2. To Promote Research, Education, and Application of Hydrogen Medicine and Facilitate Relevant Technological Development
3. To Promote Communication and Collaboration Between Domestic and International Medical Facilities and Associations for Molecular Hydrogen and Treatment Application
4. To Promote Review and Establishment of Guidelines and Regulations on Hydrogen Medicine
5. To Organize Conferences and Seminars on Hydrogen Medicine
6. To Release the Official Structure, Scientific Publications, and Code of Conduct Relating to Hydrogen Medicine

Join us here